PRAISE FOR *GETTING PAST YOUR PAST*

"Francine Shapiro's discovery of EMDR is one of the most important breakthroughs in the history of psychotherapy. Having used it as part of my practice for the past 15 years, I—and many of my patients—still marvel at the depth and speed with which it can help heal and change the minds and brains, and even bodily symptoms of people who have been locked in, and suffering from trauma, often for decades. *Getting Past Your Past* is a wonderful place to begin to understand how mental healing can occur, filled with case histories of people who are so transformed that these accounts may seem exaggerated. They are not. This book has all the sobriety of a master clinician who has worked in the field of trauma for decades, and is clear, serious, helpful, while it shares with the reader a method of healing trauma that has already helped millions."

—*Norman Doidge, MD, author of* The Brain That Changes Itself

"Francine Shapiro has given a life-transforming gift to the world by her rigorous development of a science-validated approach to soothing the suffering of our small and large life traumas. Our experiences are remembered in networks of interconnected neural patterns that can later create maladaptive ways of thinking, feeling, and behaving that may form prisons of the mind, forcing us to live in automatic ways we may believe we cannot change. Yet how we focus the mind can actually change the very structure of the brain itself. The key is to know how to use our awareness to create this important healing. Through case examples and clearly articulated instructions within *Getting Past Your Past*, our skillful guide takes us through the powerful and practical steps, derived from the treatment of literally millions of people, that can transform trauma into triumph. Explore this book with someone you love...beginning with yourself!"

—*Daniel J. Siegel, MD, clinical professor of psychiatry at UCLA School of Medicine and author of* The Developing Mind and Mindsight

"Real people, real-life stories, and real emotional healing of past hurts and traumas! In this book, Dr. Shapiro offers a collection of self-help techniques facilitating emotional healing based on EMDR therapy, used

by thousands of clinicians and proven successful. Her true stories depict
how stressful, painful, or traumatic experiences influence our lives and
block our potential—and how they can be changed and even resolved.
An eye-opener to the layperson!"

—*Ruth Colvin, recipient of the Presidential*
Medal of Freedom, cofounder of ProLiteracy

"I am forever indebted to Francine Shapiro and EMDR therapy, which
helped me to heal from a terrifying panic disorder. People in pain will
now be able to read this groundbreaking book and understand how
disturbing memories can be reprocessed. Our lives can become joyful
instead of fearful. We can live in the present instead of the past."

—*Priscilla Warner, author of* Learning to Breathe
and coauthor of The Faith Club

"It appears that Dr. Francine Shapiro has discovered a profound linkage
between the mind and body so that each might be healed. These stories
of the rebalancing and revivifying of our dynamic nature reminds
us that there are successful approaches to healing that are presently
offering remarkable cures."

—*Stephen and Ondrea Levine, authors of* Who Dies?:
An Investigation of Conscious Living and Conscious Dying

"In *Getting Past Your Past*, Dr. Francine Shapiro, the developer of
EMDR and one of the leading clinical innovators in psychotherapy,
translates her groundbreaking method into practical suggestions for
those who have been stuck in past events from which they have been
unable to free themselves. Eminently readable, Dr. Shapiro has written a
volume that is a wonderful resource for those in psychotherapy, as well
as those seeking to help themselves. This is a valuable companion for
anyone who seeks an understanding of how the past can be carried in
our memory networks influencing how we perceive the world, as well
as offering practical strategies for growth."

—*Jeffrey J. Magnavita, PhD, ABPP, past president of the*
Division of Psychotherapy of the American Psychological
Association and founder of the Unified Psychotherapy Project

"I am grateful to Francine Shapiro for having written *Getting Past Your Past*, a lucid and practical book for transforming people's lives and helping them to savor living in the moment. EMDR is a powerfully effective treatment for overcoming the traumatic imprints of the past."

—*Bessel van der Kolk MD, medical director of the Trauma Center at the Justice Resource Institute, director of the National Complex Trauma Treatment Network, and professor of psychiatry at Boston University School of Medicine*

"*Getting Past Your Past* provides readers with powerful new insights to understand how traumas and disturbances of all kinds disrupt human potential, and how they can deal with their own distress. Through well-chosen case studies the reader shares the profound experiences of a wide range of individuals and learns the EMDR treatment strategies that have enabled clients to strip "visceral" feelings from memories as a turning point on their path to self-regulation and personal safety."

—*Stephen W. Porges, PhD, professor of psychiatry and director of the Brain-Body Center at the University of Illinois at Chicago and author of* The Polyvagal Theory: Neurophysiological Foundations of Emotions, Attachment, Communication, and Self-Regulation

"In *Getting Past Your Past*, Francine Shapiro takes her innovative therapy, EMDR, to people everywhere, making the insights and strategies of EMDR treatment available to a broad audience. The transformation of EMDR treatment strategies into self-help techniques is yet another step in Shapiro's journey to make healing from trauma available to all. This book will be a valuable resource for therapists and clients alike, as well as for the many individuals who struggle with the effects of painful life experiences but who do not seek formal treatment."

—*Laura S. Brown, PhD, ABPP past president of APA Division of Trauma Psychology and director of Fremont Community Therapy Project*

"Are you painfully enslaved by emotional roadblocks and/or poor relationship choices? Unprocessed memories could be the problem... and EMDR could be the answer. EMDR is a powerful, scientifically validated process that has helped millions of people reclaim their freedom. In *Getting Past Your Past*, Francine Shapiro makes her practical methods available to the public for the first time. This is self-help at its finest."

—Jeffrey K. Zeig, PhD, director of the Milton Erickson Foundation, and director of the Evolution of Psychotherapy Conference

"This self-help book is a cause for tremendous optimism. With EMDR the world finally has a therapy against the damaging effects of trauma, one that is scientifically proven to be effective and quick, low-cost, and widely applicable in a range of settings and cultural milieus. The future of the human potential—and the world—looks so much brighter for Francine Shapiro's discovery of EMDR."

—Rolf C. Carriere, former UN development professional and UNICEF representative in five Asian countries

GETTING PAST YOUR PAST

TAKE CONTROL OF YOUR LIFE
WITH SELF-HELP TECHNIQUES
FROM EMDR THERAPY

FRANCINE SHAPIRO, PhD

RODALE.

To my beloved husband,
Bob Welch

© 2012 by Francine Shapiro, PhD

All rights reserved. No part of this publication may be reproduced or transmitted in any form or by any means, electronic or mechanical, including photocopying, recording, or any other information storage and retrieval system, without the written permission of the publisher.

Rodale books may be purchased for business or promotional use or for special sales. For information, please write to:
Special Markets Department, Rodale Inc., 733 Third Avenue, New York, NY 10017

Printed in the United States of America
Rodale Inc. makes every effort to use acid-free ⊗ recycled paper ♻

Book design by Christina Gaugler

Library of Congress Cataloging-in-Publication Data is on file with the publisher.

ISBN 978–1–60961–995–4   paperback

Distributed to the trade by Macmillan

21   paperback

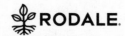

We inspire and enable people to improve their lives and the world around them.
rodalebooks.com

CONTENTS

CHAPTER 1: Running on Automatic 1

CHAPTER 2: Mind, Brain and What Matters 19

CHAPTER 3: Is It the Climate or the Weather? 44

CHAPTER 4: What's Running Your Show? 70

CHAPTER 5: The Hidden Landscape 95

CHAPTER 6: I Would If I Could, But I Can't 120

CHAPTER 7: The Brain, Body and Mind Connection 151

CHAPTER 8: What Do You Want from Me? 181

CHAPTER 9: A Part of the Whole 215

CHAPTER 10: From Stressed to Better Than Well 247

CHAPTER 11: Bringing It Home 275

Acknowledgments 303

Appendix A—Glossary and Self-Help Techniques,
Audio Recordings, and Personal Table 306

Appendix B—Choosing a Clinician; EMDR Therapy and
Training Resources; and EMDR-Humanitarian
Assistance Programs (HAP) 310

Appendix C—EMDR: Trauma Research Findings
and Further Reading 315

Appendix D—Selected References 321

Index 339

RUNNING
ON AUTOMATIC

W*hy would a beautiful, intelligent woman keep picking the wrong men, and then when they try to break up with her, throw herself on the floor clutching their legs, begging them not to leave?*

Ben is a successful businessman. Why is he hit with anxiety whenever he has to make a presentation?

Stacey has been trying one therapist after another for years to discover why she has an almost constant feeling of dread, fears of abandonment and an eating disorder. Strangest of all, she has repeated images of the color red and a candle. It makes no sense to her, but it has been going on for as long as she can remember.

Interestingly, there is a simple explanation for their problems that involves how the brain itself functions. In this book, we will explore both the reasons for suffering and what we can do about it.

WHY WE SUFFER

The truth is we all suffer at one time or another. Situations arise all the time that affect us negatively. But when we continue to have pain long after the experience itself has passed, it is because the hardwiring of our brains influences our minds. Let's try the following experiment so you can see for yourself. I'll give a single sentence and you just notice the first thing that pops into your mind:

Roses are red

_____

The odds are that the first thing to come up was: Violets are blue. For people born in the United States, it's basically the equivalent of a knee-jerk response. This is an important concept, since mental responses are based on physical reactions. Your brain is programmed to respond in the same way as the rest of your body. Regardless of age or gender, when your knee is hit in a certain way your leg will jerk. Similarly, regardless of intention, your mind also reacts automatically. For instance, when is the last time you heard that rhyme? You probably learned it in childhood. So, if you don't live with young children, it was likely many, many years ago. But it came up automatically nonetheless. These types of automatic responses can be wonderful and useful, and show the power of our minds, but they don't always serve us.

Take a look at the sentences themselves. Your response to "Roses are red" wasn't a critical evaluation of its meaning. Your mind just moved along with a response as if it was true. But roses aren't always red. They are also yellow, pink, purple and most any color you can think of. However, that unexamined sentence looks just fine at first glance. And how about the second one: Violets are blue. Are they really? No, actually they are purple. But the line will come up whether it's true or not. Now, probably the sentence didn't cause you any kind of distress. But that same type of automatic response also causes a wide range of problems that disrupt happiness, families and communities. The same mind/brain processes that allow us to recognize a rhyme, or sing along with a tune we haven't heard in 20 years, are the ones that can also drown us in the misery of anxiety, depression, heartache and at times physical pain.

The nursery rhyme has even more to offer. Remember the line that comes after "Violets are blue"? "Sugar is sweet and so are you." Lovely sentiment, and it also comes to mind automatically. But as we all know, while sugar is surely sweet, people are lots more complicated. Everyone is a mixture of sweet, sour and every flavor and variation under the sun. At some point, everyone is angry, sad, jealous, bitter, hurt, insecure, happy or sweet. And when we are, we act accordingly. One moment we cherish the one we are with and cover them with kisses. A day later we may explode and yell at them in frustration. So, basically, some of what we've learned growing up is true, but just as with all the other experiences we've had through childhood, other things are not. Often as youngsters we can't tell the difference, and what we take to be real—such as believing we are inferior because we are bullied or rejected, or thinking we are responsible for our parents' divorce—are really just misperceptions. Nevertheless, these experiences can have effects that come up automatically throughout the rest of our lives, outside our conscious control.

Every experience we've had in our lives has become a building block in our inner world, governing our reactions to everything and every person we encounter. When we "learn" something, the experience is physically stored within networks of brain cells called "neurons." These networks actually form our unconscious mind, determining how our brain interprets the world around us and governing how we feel from moment to moment. These memories include experiences that took place years ago, and our conscious mind is often unaware that they have any impact on us at all. But since the memories are physically stored in the brain, they can pop up outside our control in response to "Roses are red," just as they color our view of every new situation we encounter. They can cause us to feel unattractive when we're not. Depressed when everyone else around us is happy. And they can leave us feeling heartsick if someone leaves us—even if we know consciously that the person is terrible for us and continuing the relationship would be a big mistake. Basically, many of the feelings and actions that undermine our happiness are symptoms that stem from this memory system that forms the unconscious.

Let's take the first case from page 1:

Why would a beautiful, intelligent woman keep picking the wrong men, and then when they try to break up with her, throw herself on the floor clutching their legs, begging them not to leave?

Justine has no problems getting boyfriends. Her problem is keeping them. Now 25 years old, she generally picks men with an "edge" who are emotionally unavailable. Then every time she gets into a relationship, she begins acting clingy and her boyfriend eventually breaks up with her. When this happens, she begins to cry hysterically, falling to her knees and putting her arms around the man's legs, pleading with him not to leave her. In therapy, the cause of this was tracked back to something that happened on a Sunday evening when she was 6 years old. Justine was living with her parents in a two-story house. On that night there was a severe thunderstorm, causing her to become very frightened. Upstairs in her bedroom, she began crying and yelling for her mommy and daddy to come to her. However, they were in the kitchen on the first floor. The storm drowned out her screams, and they didn't hear her. They never came to her rescue and she eventually cried herself to sleep.

How could something as common as this be responsible for her problems? All of us have experienced loud storms sometime in childhood, but only some of us will remain negatively affected by it. We'll go into the detailed reasons for this in later chapters. For now, it's sufficient to know that when negative reactions and behaviors in the present can be tracked directly back to an earlier memory, we define those memories as "unprocessed"—meaning that they are stored in the brain in a way that still holds the emotions, physical sensations and beliefs that were experienced earlier in life. That stormy night Justine was intensely frightened as a child, and had the belief that she was in danger. Her parents didn't come when she cried for them, which also gave her the feeling that she would be abandoned if she really needed them. This memory, stored in her brain with the intense fear she experienced at 6 years old, is stimulated whenever a boyfriend breaks up with her. At this point, she no longer functions as a mature and successful 25-year-old, but instead as a frightened little girl left alone in the dark. We can see the connection, given that the storm and a breakup are both associated with aloneness and abandonment. As such, she unconsciously experiences the breakup as "being in danger."

We experience these types of connections all the time. It's generally the reason for all of the characteristics we love or hate in ourselves and the people around us. It's simply part of the way the brain functions in order to make sense of the world. But identifying the memory connections is just the first step in changing how we think, act or feel. It's not just understanding where something comes from, but also knowing what to do about it that's important. In the course of this book we will be exploring how to identify the memories that underlie personal and relationship problems; what we can do to help manage them on our own; and how to recognize when further professional help would be useful.

We'll also explore the workings of the mind—the intricate connections that form our consciousness—through stories contributed by some of the more than 70,000 clinicians worldwide who practice a form of therapy known as Eye Movement Desensitization and Reprocessing (EMDR). Millions of people have been helped by the therapy over the past 20 years, and many of them are giving detailed reports in this book in order to help "demystify" the change process. As research has shown, major changes can take place within even one EMDR reprocessing session. The clients' reports allow us a "window into the brain," since the connections they made answer so many questions about why we react to the world in different ways.

EMDR therapy targets the unprocessed memories that contain the negative emotions, sensations and beliefs. By activating the brain's information processing system (which will be explained in Chapter 2), the old memories can then be "digested." Meaning what is useful is learned, what's useless is discarded, and the memory is now stored in a way that is no longer damaging. For instance, Justine's clinician focused on the thunderstorm along with the feeling she had of being alone and in danger. Once the memory of the thunderstorm was processed, the childhood sensations of terror disappeared and were replaced by the feeling of safety, and the belief that as an adult she could take care of herself. Along with that, the boyfriend problem resolved as her new sense of self resulted in her making different romantic choices. Of course there would be more memories that might have to be dealt with if Justine's parents had been generally abusive or neglectful. But regardless of the number of memories involved, basically we are entering into the person's "unconscious" mind with this form of therapy, in a way that can allow insights, connections and change to occur rapidly within the reprocessing sessions.

WHAT IS THE UNCONSCIOUS MIND?

When most people think of the unconscious, they think of psychoanalysis and movies that involve a Freudian view of psychic conflicts, and symbolic dreams and gestures. From the psychoanalytic perspective it generally takes years of talk therapy and "working through" to gain insight and mastery over forces that are hidden from view. This form of therapy can have great value. But Freud published first in 1900, and many things have changed since then. In the past century there have been new advances in neurobiological technologies that have expanded our understanding of what these "forces" actually are. The examination of the unconscious we are dealing with in this book is one that is based on the workings of the brain itself. Through an understanding of how experiences lay the physical groundwork for our emotional and physical reactions, we can determine how our "stuck" points and knee-jerk mental responses came about and what to do about them.

For instance, let's take the second case:

Ben is a successful businessman. Why is he hit with anxiety whenever he has to make a presentation? Here's how he described it:

"As long as I can remember, I've had anxiety about doing any performance in front of a group of people. My palms sweat, my voice becomes unpredictable, my heart beats fast and I have thoughts like, 'I'm an idiot. I can't do this. Everyone will hate me.' It sometimes felt as though my life was at risk. Sounds ridiculous, but it was so true. As I went through school, there were many times in the normal course of events when I had to make public presentations. In my professional career the same thing happened. I always made it through these events, but not happily. In fact, I suffered before and after every event, and tediously went over every detail with my loved ones, which, as you might imagine, did not delight them. No matter what I tried, nothing seemed to fix this problem. I tried many types of therapy. Sometimes it seemed a little better, but it always came roaring back."

Ben entered into EMDR therapy and used a variety of procedures that we'll learn in this book to identify the source of his problem and change his reactions. Here's what he discovered: "It turns out the cause was something that happened to me when I was no more than 3½ years old. I was walking with my grandfather on his farm in western North Carolina. My memory here is as if I was looking up, like a very small child. I don't remember chattering away to my grandfather, but if family stories can be trusted, I probably was. We met a strange man on the road. He was old, bent, angry looking, with very hairy nostrils. He said to my grandfather in his mountain drawl, 'Well, howdy, if I had a youn-gun' talked as much as that un, I'd drown him in the creek.' I slipped behind my grandfather's denim-covered leg, peered up the man's nostrils and shut up. I knew that unwanted kittens were in fact 'drowned in the creek.' It did not seem safe to chatter in front of strangers."

So, this child's moment of terror set the groundwork for his problem. The memory became stored in his brain and set him up for failure: "I did my first book report in third grade in front of my beloved Ms. Kneenor, a young, pretty, first-year teacher. I loved Ms. Kneenor, and was very proud of the fact that my book report was three pages long. I had worked very hard on it. I had also developed a slight stutter, which lasted all of about six months before leaving as mysteriously as it began. My parents had handled this pretty well, and I wasn't aware of being self-conscious about it. I had daydreams of Ms. K praising me and telling the class what a great report I had done. Instead, Ms. K stayed in the back of the room in out-of-control laughter during my whole report. As I shuffled through my report, the stutter getting worse as I went, I thought, 'I'm an idiot.'

Then two years later I was recruited at the last minute to do a part in a school play. I was in the middle of the first act when I forgot my lines. I stood in the middle of the stage stock-still. I thought, 'Everyone will hate me. I have ruined the play. I'm an idiot.'"

Notice that Ben had these same thoughts going through his mind 40 years later when he needed to make a presentation at work: "I'm an idiot. I can't do this. Everyone will hate me." He had no idea before EMDR therapy why he was feeling and thinking that way. He did not have a visual image of his grandfather's farm, or the book report, or the school play—he just had the feelings and thoughts that went along with it. This was an automatic response to an external "trigger," just as much as "Roses are red" causes "Violets are blue."

Nothing exists in a vacuum. Reactions that seem irrational are often exactly that. But irrational doesn't mean that there is no reason for them. It means that the responses come from a part of our brain that is not governed by the rational mind. The automatic reactions that control our emotions come from neural associations within our memory networks that are independent of our higher reasoning power. That's why you can watch in amazement as you do something you know you'll regret later, or get drawn to the wrong people, or feel hurt by someone you have no respect for, or yell at a loved one with little reason, or feel powerless to shake a depression brought on by something that seems inconsequential. It's irrational but understandable and, more important, it's fixable. While genetics play an important role, in general, the basis of the suffering is the way our memories of past experiences are stored in the brain, and this can be changed. Happily, appropriately stored memories are also the basis of joy and mental health. Later on, we'll explore more about how the brain and memories work.

WE'RE ALL IN THIS TOGETHER

We are all on a continuum of suffering and happiness, of sickness and health, of families who contributed to our problems and those who were supportive and loving. Likewise, the kinds of experiences we have encountered range from the usual ones of childhood humiliations, failures, rejection and arguments to the major events needed to diagnose posttraumatic stress disorder (PTSD), such as major accidents, physical, sexual or emotional abuse, combat, or natural disasters. In addition, for someone to be diagnosed with PTSD, they have to have symptoms such as intrusive thoughts, sleep disturbances such as nightmares or recurrent dreams, anxiety, "hyperarousal" where they are extremely alert for danger and may jump at loud noises, or "numbing" where they feel shut down and disconnected. They also try to stay away from reminders of the event, but thoughts of it keep popping up anyway.

People with PTSD clearly have the negative experience stored in their brain in a way that is highly disturbing. So when a combat veteran with PTSD thinks back to an event that happened in Iraq or Afghanistan three years ago, he can feel it in his body, with the thoughts and images that were there at the time of the event. The veteran who came back from the Vietnam War can think of something that happened more than 30 years ago, and the same thing happens. A Marine who has gone through many tours of duty and witnessed many casualties can be haunted by one particular death. When he thinks about it he can feel the same helplessness, pain, sorrow and anger he felt at the time. And he responds to the world around him with those emotions.

Likewise, if someone who was raped a year ago or molested 50 years ago has PTSD, the past is present. When they think of the incident, it can feel as though it's happening all over again, or they can be fearful and anxious when around certain people or places. But regardless of how long ago something happened, and regardless of how long symptoms have been there, it doesn't need to be permanent. The research is clear on that. Also important, although a major trauma such as robbery or violence is needed to give a formal diagnosis of PTSD, a number of recent studies have demonstrated that everyday life experiences, such as relationship problems or unemployment, can produce just as many, and sometimes even more, symptoms of PTSD.

This has important implications for all of us. It shows that there is no clear separation between kinds of events, nor is there a clear separation between symptoms. Similar to those who suffer from PTSD, we all have had the experience of feeling anxious, fearful, jumpy or shut off from others, thoughts we can't get out of our heads, guilt, or disturbing dreams. Sometimes those reactions are based on a current situation and we need to think about it and get the information needed to handle it. For others, the symptoms go away when the situation changes. But for many of us, these feelings occur often or for no apparent reason. These are generally signs that there are underlying unprocessed memories causing them. These memories can be identified and treated. So it's useful to remember that whatever the persistent negative emotion, belief or behavior that has been bothering you, it's not the cause of suffering—*it's the symptom*. The likely cause is the memory that's pushing it. Our memories are the basis of both negative symptoms and of mental health. The key difference is the way the memories are stored in the brain. If they are unprocessed, they can cause us to overreact or act in a way that hurts us or those around us. If they are "processed," we are able to react in ways that serve our loved ones and ourselves well.

WHY ME?

Those of us who were raised by parents who were unsupportive or abusive have an idea of the kinds of experiences that might be causing some of our problems. Others have read stories of really disturbed families and messed-up childhoods, and believe "That's not me. I had a good family so it makes no sense for me to feel the way I do." However, sometimes even with the most supportive family members who believe they are doing the best for us, we can find ourselves locked in a web of symptoms and pain that we don't understand. And sometimes the search for answers in therapy can lead us astray, because the clinician does not have a clear idea about how memory works. For instance, let's take a look at our third example:

Why does Stacey have an almost constant feeling of dread, fears of abandonment and an eating disorder? Strangest of all, she has repeated images of the color red and a candle. It makes no sense to her, but it has been going on for as long as she can remember.

Stacey tried one therapist after another for years. There are more than 100 different kinds of therapy, and each therapist brings a personal perspective, which also changes the way the treatment is applied. Sometimes it's difficult for people to find the right treatment—or the right therapist. Also, clinical situations can be complicated, because sometimes a childhood event is so disturbing that it can completely overwhelm the brain's natural ability to process it, and it's either not stored at all or becomes completely cut off so the person can't remember it. That was one of Stacey's problems. After years of therapy with little change in symptoms, she arrived at a therapist who tried a variety of avenues and also got no results. Since Stacey had no idea where the problems came from, and had abandonment issues, intimacy problems, eating difficulties, panic and anxiety, her clinician said to her, "It really sounds like you have been sexually abused." In addition, because she had recurrent images of the color red and a candle, he suggested that maybe it was ritual abuse because those images would fit right into satanic worship ceremonies. As you can imagine, that made her anxiety even worse. So for two years, they probed her life story, trying without success to find memories of ritual abuse.

Since she was still suffering, Stacey tried another therapist where she learned about EMDR. Because she didn't have recall of anything she consciously felt was connected to the feelings of dread, anxiety, fears of abandonment and her eating disorder, the therapist targeted the symptoms that could most directly lead to the underlying memory: the image of the color red and a candle. After the appropriate preparation, during the memory processing procedures, images from her childhood emerged and she saw herself at about 5 years old. It was her birthday. Her daddy gave her a scented candle for her room and then they went off in the car to her birthday luncheon. As they are driving along singing together, a car runs a stoplight and crashes into them, killing her father. So if her father died next to her on the way to her birthday luncheon, the symptoms become explainable. As you can see, from this you could easily develop eating problems, abandonment issues and persistent anxiety.

But sometimes memories can be misleading, because they can simply be images that conform to the feelings we have. For instance, children can believe that something bad happened to them because they heard a story or saw something on television. Think of all the children who develop nightmares after watching frightening movies. Was Stacey really in the car when her father was killed? Stacey knew that her father had died in a car accident but she'd had no memory of being with him. You don't know unless you get confirmation. She called up her mother and asked, "Mom, is it true? Was I with Dad when he died?" Her mother said, "Well, yes dear, you were, but we thought you didn't want to talk about it because you never mentioned it." So even though Stacey had a very loving mother who wanted to protect her and no direct memory of her father's death, she had years of symptoms that seemed totally irrational. Now they made sense. And more important, they disappeared after the memory was processed.

It's important to remember that we don't have to undergo a major trauma such as a father's death or a car accident to develop symptoms that last for years. For instance, Janice came in for therapy with a very long history of taking too many antacids. At this point it was life threatening because she was taking them so often that they were practically ripping up her stomach. She also had no memory of why it had started; she only knew that she was horrified of getting sick to her stomach. The clinician used the EMDR procedures you'll be learning to find the source of these feelings. What Janice then remembered was being in grade school when the girl next to her in class vomited. Trying to stop herself, the girl put her hand over her mouth and the vomit went sideways into Janice's hair. Janice went running out of the room feeling panicky, humiliated and unclean. This was the memory at the bottom of the antacid abuse. After processing the memory, she no longer felt the need for them.

So if there is a symptom, the message is that there is usually some experience that caused or is contributing to it. Something happened, whether we consciously remember it or not. Although we have come to rely heavily on pills for feelings of well-being, many times they only mask the symptoms. The cause of these problems is not typically an innate neurological difficulty or purely biochemical. Of course our genetic makeup plays an important role and can cause us to react strongly to certain experiences. Sometimes we can inherit predispositions to a variety of vulnerable states, such as depression or anxiety.

However, even in these cases, certain types of life experiences are generally needed to cause distress. Basically, our genetic makeup combines with our experiences in ways that can make life go on "automatic pilot."

The other message is that just because the symptoms are long lasting or severe, it doesn't necessarily mean there was a major trauma. Even seemingly minor events from an adult perspective can be the cause. The bottom line is that from the vantage point of a child, it felt traumatic at the time and the memory was locked into the brain. These experiences may have happened long ago, and we may not recognize how much they actually affected us. But the negative emotions, behaviors, beliefs and sensations that cause chronic problems generally can be tracked back to these unprocessed memories. In that way the past stays present. This book will provide techniques that can help you make sense of symptoms and identify their cause. We'll also demonstrate ways in which your thoughts, feelings and reactions can be transformed, lowering distress and increasing confidence and comfort.

THE GOALS OF THIS BOOK

There are thousands of things that send us looking for answers, whether in books or through therapy. Some people simply need information to deal with a new event in their lives. Others recognize that something is blocking them. They are being pushed into doing things they don't want to do, or they are being prevented from doing things they know would benefit them. This book is about understanding the "Why" in your life, and in those around you. More important, it's also about understanding what you can do about it. We all have moments of pain and uncertainty. It's not a question of "Will I suffer sometime in my life?" Rather, it's how long and in how many ways. Some of us move rapidly through certain kinds of pain, but not through others. Some of us are joyful, while others feel joy rarely or not at all. This book is about understanding why we are who we are, and learning what we can do about pain and negative reactions that don't serve us. It's also about identifying and opening the blocks to feelings of happiness and well-being. By using a number of the techniques, you can decide for yourself how to make the best choices for your future.

I also want to emphasize that while we often find that experiences from childhood are the root cause of many psychological problems, this book is not about "blame." As a child in a world of adults, everyone had experiences of not being in control, being ignored or feeling less important than other people. We'll explore in later chapters why psychological symptoms and problems develop for some and not for others. But it is important to remember that all of these things occurred before we had any choices or power. As children, we didn't ask for what happened to us. And whatever kind of parenting we had, our parents also are who they are because of their own life experiences, including the way they were raised. Basically, if we want to assign blame, we generally have to go back through generations. Nevertheless, even the longest negative patterns can be broken. As responsible adults with sufficient knowledge, we have the power to take control of ourselves.

As we identify the forces at work in our lives, we can better understand what makes us tick—and also better understand those around us. We are all dealing with unconscious processes and memories that govern our feelings and actions. Ultimately, the question is: What do we do about it? For instance, Joe came to see me because although he was unhappy at work and realized it was a bad fit, he couldn't bring himself to change jobs. As we explored his feelings, he said that he'd always had the sense that "I can't go after and get what I want." Using the EMDR procedures, we were able to discover and process the memory that was holding him back. Joe remembered himself as a little boy playing with a ball at the top of the stairs. His mother saw him and told him not to go down the steps. But the ball rolled down, and in his excitement he ran after the ball. His mother came after him, grabbed him by the arm and started spanking him: punishing him for going after what he wanted. That simple event locked in the negative feelings and the belief connected with it for the next 30 years.

Another thing to keep in mind is that this is not an example of an abusive childhood. Joe's mother was most often kind and loving, but she reacted out of her own fear that disobeying her would hurt him. Her parenting style was forged by her own upbringing. It was simply one event in Joe's lifetime. But individual memories can get stored in a way that leaves the negative emotions, physical sensations and beliefs unchanged regardless of whatever else happens in a person's life.

Since memories form the basis of our personality characteristics and how we respond in the world, we'll explore ways to identify the memories that may be at the root of both emotional and physical pain. Chapters in this book will also explore problems involving self-esteem, depression, anxiety, addictions, relationships and parenting issues, job problems, loss and even physical conditions. You'll also learn specific techniques you can use to help deal with each of these issues, and guidelines for knowing when further assistance is needed. It's important to remember that while unprocessed memories are often the source of symptoms and pain, processed memories are the basis of mental health. So we'll also explore some of the procedures that can boost your sense of empowerment that have been used by Olympic athletes and others to achieve their performance goals.

The bottom line is that regardless of how we were brought up, we are not victims and our problems are not a sign of weakness. Some of the most gloried heroes, those who risk themselves for others, who faced all odds to bring someone to safety, are the ones who can needlessly suffer the most internally through guilt about who they couldn't save or what they couldn't accomplish. When we recognize that we are being held back in life, the question for each of us is "What do I do about it?"

MIND, BRAIN AND WHAT MATTERS

W e all interact with the world around us with brains and bodies that have more similarities than differences. Most people are trying to do their best for themselves and their families. Nevertheless, despite these commonalities, something often gets in the way. The reasons for this will be easier to recognize after we set the groundwork for understanding the basis of the procedures we'll be covering in the rest of the book. Genetic factors can certainly be involved. But how we view the world and interact with others is largely based upon our individual life experiences. These are stored in memory networks that are the basis of our perceptions, attitudes and behavior. And these networks link up similar events.

For instance, if someone asks me to name several different fruits, I have no problem doing that. In my mind, they are associated within a memory network . . . apples, oranges, pears, blueberries. If I see an apple, I can easily recognize it as a fruit because I've seen one before. What I am experiencing at any given time becomes linked into my memory network of past experiences so that I can make sense of it. However, if a child has never seen an apple before, she might not know what to do with it. It's red and it's round: Is it a ball?

Awareness of anything in the outside world comes through our senses (sight, smell, touch, hearing, taste) into working memory. This automatically links into a wide range of memory networks in the brain to help us understand what we are perceiving.

This process is going on for all of us all the time. Even the words on this page have to link up to your memory networks so that you can understand what you're reading. Everybody you see, everyone you interact with, all of the experiences that you have in the present and your perceptions of those present experiences link up to your memory networks in order for you to make sense of them. Those memory networks have all of your other already stored experiences within them. They become the basis of how you're feeling, thinking and behaving in the moment. So, how you respond to the people in your life, and how they respond to you, is based just as much on past experiences as it is on whatever either of you does or says in the present.

WHY TIME DOESN'T HEAL ALL WOUNDS

If we cut ourselves, unless there is an obstacle, we tend to heal. If we remove the block, the body goes back to healing. That's why we're willing to let ourselves be cut open during surgery. We expect incisions to heal.

The brain is part of the body. In addition to the millions of memory networks I've just described, we all have hardwired into our brains a mechanism—an information processing system—for healing. It is geared to take any sort of emotional turmoil to a level of mental health or what I call a level of *adaptive resolution*. This means a resolution that includes the useful information that allows us to be more fit for survival in our lives. The information processing system is meant to make connections to what is useful, and let go of the rest.

Here's how it works: Imagine that you've had an argument with a coworker. You can feel upset, angry or fearful with all the physical reactions that go along with these different emotions. You can also have negative thoughts about the person and yourself. You might imagine how you'd like to exact revenge, but let's hope you resist those behaviors; among other things they would probably get you fired. So you walk away. You think about it. You talk about it. You go to sleep and maybe dream about it. And the next day you might not feel so bad. You've basically "digested" the experience and now have a better sense of what to do. That's the brain's information processing system taking a disturbing experience and allowing learning to take place. Much of it goes on during rapid eye movement (REM) sleep. Scientists believe that during this stage of sleep the brain processes wishes, survival information and the learning that took place that day. Basically, whatever is important to us. The bottom line is that the brain is hardwired to do that.

After uninterrupted information processing, the memory of the argument has generally linked up with more useful information already stored in your brain. This can include past experiences you've had with this coworker and others. You may now be able to say, "Oh, that's just the way John is. I've handled something like this before with him, and it came out fine." As these other memories link up with the current disturbing incident, your experience of the event changes. You learn what is useful from the argument and your brain lets go of what's not. Because the negative feelings and the self-talk are no longer useful, they're gone. But what you needed to learn remains, and now your brain stores the memory of the event in a form where it is able to successfully guide you in the future.

As a result, you have a better sense of what you're supposed to do. You can talk to your coworker without the intense emotional turmoil you had the day before. That's the brain's adaptive information processing system taking a disturbing experience and allowing learning to take place. It's doing just what it's geared to do.

Sadly, disturbing experiences, whether major traumas or other kinds of upsetting events, can overwhelm the system. When that happens, the intense emotional and physical disturbance caused by the situation prevents the information processing system from making the internal connections needed to take it to a resolution. Instead, the memory of the situation becomes stored in the brain as you experienced it. What you saw and felt, the image, the emotions, the physical sensations and the thoughts become encoded in memory in their original, unprocessed form. So, whenever you see the coworker you argued with, rather than being able to have a calm chat, the anger or fear comes flooding back. You may try to manage your feelings out of self-preservation, but whenever the person appears, your distress goes up.

When reactions such as these refuse to go away in the present, it's often because they are also linking into unprocessed memories from the past. These unconscious connections occur automatically. For instance, your immediate dislike of a person you just met may come from memories of someone in some way similar who hurt you before. Also, consider the case of a woman who was raped. Years later, she is in bed with someone she knows is a very loving partner. But when he touches her in a certain way, her emotions and body respond automatically. The terror and feelings of powerlessness she had during the rape flood her. If the information processing system did not function properly after the attack, a touch similar to the rapist's can link into the memory network and "trigger" the emotions and the physical sensations that are part of that stored unprocessed memory.

The disrupted information processing system has stored the memory in isolation—unintegrated within the more general memory networks. It can't change since it is unable to link up with anything more useful and adaptive. That's why time doesn't heal all wounds, and you may still feel anger, resentment, pain, sorrow or a number of other emotions about events that took place years ago. They are frozen in time, and the unprocessed memories can become the foundation for emotional, and sometimes physical, problems. Even though you might not have had a major trauma in your life, research has shown that other kinds of life experiences can cause the same types of problems. And since the memory connections happen automatically, below conscious level, you may have no idea what's really running your show.

THE PLAN OF ACTION

As we proceed, you'll learn how to make sense of negative reactions you or a loved one may be having in a wide range of situations. You'll also learn exercises and techniques to identify unprocessed memories that are causing these reactions and ways to immediately deal with disturbing emotions, thoughts and sensations. These steps you can take are based on new knowledge about how the brain works. The good news is that they can free you from bonds that may have held you back in relationships, work and general happiness.

Most of the procedures and stories you'll find in this book come from a therapy called EMDR. So in this chapter I'll introduce you to EMDR, and then show you how the different kinds of memory connections that it has revealed can be the basis for your own unhappiness. We'll also see how these connections can be transformed into a foundation of joy, peace and well-being. In the following chapters, you'll begin learning some of the techniques that thousands of clinicians are using worldwide. They help people with a variety of different issues that may also apply to you.

EMDR THERAPY

Where does EMDR therapy come from? How did it develop? Why does it work?

EMDR stands for Eye Movement Desensitization and Reprocessing. It started because of a discovery I made about eye movements. I was walking in the park one day in 1987 and suddenly realized that some disturbing thoughts I was having had disappeared. I don't remember what I was thinking about. But they were the kind of niggling, nagging thoughts about a current problem that you generally have to do something deliberate about to get to change. When I brought the thoughts back, they didn't have the same "charge" to them. They simply didn't bother me anymore.

I was surprised and wondered what caused this reaction. So as I walked along, I started to pay careful attention. I noticed that when that kind of thought came to mind, my eyes started moving very rapidly back and forth diagonally in a certain way. Then the thought shifted from my consciousness. When I brought it back again, it had lost its power. This fascinated me, so I started doing it deliberately. I brought up something that bothered me, and I started doing the eye movements. The same thing happened. My feelings changed.

Over the years, many have wondered why I noticed my thoughts changing after the eye movements. I suppose it's an example of a chance discovery—and many years of preparation. Luckily, I'd been using my own mind and body as a "laboratory" for the previous ten years after a bout with cancer. The doctors had said, "It's gone, but some people get it back. We don't know why, and we don't know who. So good luck." At that point it struck me as ironic that we were putting men on the moon, but didn't know how to deal with our own minds and bodies. The field of psychoneuroimmunology—studying the effects of stress on our immune systems—had just begun to open up based on the work of Norman Cousins and others. So I decided to search for whatever practical information might be available and get it out to the general public.

Over the following years, I investigated dozens of workshops, studied with numerous teachers, and entered a formal psychology doctoral program. So, when my thoughts changed unexpectedly, it caught my attention. I believed I'd stumbled onto the brain's natural healing process. This worked right into what I'd been exploring for the past ten years— how the mind and body were connected. I wondered whether my observation about eye movements was related in some way to the processes that occur during REM sleep. Since eye movements happened spontaneously during that period of dream sleep, and we often awaken feeling better about situations in our lives, maybe they have the same effect when we are awake.

After I found that I could change the feelings connected to my thoughts by deliberately using the eye movements, I wondered if it would work for other people. So I tried it with everyone I knew who was willing. I asked them to think of something that bothered them. Not surprisingly, they all had some situation they could focus on—a fight with a family member, a problem at work, a wrong decision they'd made. I would begin by asking them to concentrate on the memory. I then had them follow my hand with their eyes for about 30 seconds to re-create the same kinds of eye movements I'd experienced. I called that a "set" of eye movements—and I asked them how they felt afterward.

Most people would start to feel better—but then their feelings would stop changing. If that happened, I'd ask them to focus on a different part of the memory or what had been said. Or I'd change the direction or speed of the eye movement. Since I was getting feedback after each set, I worked through trial and error with about 70 people until the results were consistent. Since the changes were happening rapidly, if someone stalled after one set I could easily explore different alternatives to start up the positive effects again.

At the end of my doctoral program, I decided to do a controlled study on my procedure for my dissertation. It seemed that the most relevant thing to deal with was old memories. I asked myself who would have the most problem with those issues. The answer seemed clearly to be sexual abuse victims and combat veterans. That brought me to working with people who had the diagnosis of posttraumatic stress disorder (PTSD).

Back in 1987, PTSD had been accepted as a diagnosis for only seven years. At that time, there were no rigorous scientific studies validating any form of therapy for this disorder, and it was considered extremely difficult to treat. So I decided to test the effectiveness of my procedure with people suffering from that disorder. The results of my randomized controlled research were published in the *Journal of Traumatic Stress* in 1989. As you can imagine, since the article described a brand-new kind of therapy that included the use of eye movements and reported very rapid benefits for trauma victims, it created a great deal of controversy. As with any field, if something does not fit into the current understanding of how things work, it raises eyebrows, hackles or both.

Why should eye movements have any effect? How can any therapy show results within just one session? One of the "fathers" of behavior therapy announced my findings as a "breakthrough" at a major conference, and others questioned how something that seemed so simple could produce such dramatic benefits. Some people wanted training in it immediately because nothing they were doing was working well for their patients with PTSD. Others insisted that no training should be given at all.

One of the advisory board members of the *Journal of Traumatic Stress*, where my first article had been published, contacted the editor and said he was sure the journal had been duped. However, since he was in charge of a PTSD program for the Department of Veterans Affairs, he attended an EMDR training program. There he targeted one of his own experiences and saw the effects. He then tried it with his patients and became convinced that it worked. And that's how the recognition of EMDR therapy has progressed since 1990. Those people who investigate it personally generally become supporters. Those who have been influenced by the early controversy remain skeptical. However, today more than 20 scientifically controlled studies of EMDR have proven its effectiveness in the treatment of traumatic and other disturbing life experiences. At this point, a wide range of organizations worldwide, including the American Psychiatric Association and the US Department of Defense, have recognized EMDR as an effective treatment for trauma.

Since I believed initially that the primary effect of the eye movements was reducing a person's emotional disturbance—what is called "desensitization" in behavior therapy—I originally called the therapy Eye Movement Desensitization. It wasn't until after my first publication in 1989 that I realized how much more could be achieved besides anxiety reduction. Altering the procedures could also offer the opportunity for insights and automatic changes in all kinds of emotions, body reactions and behaviors. Beliefs about oneself, others and the world could change, opening up new possibilities for the future. It became clear that by further changing my methods I could ensure that the memories I targeted were fully reprocessed—connected with other memories, reorganized and stored in a better way. Therefore, after further developing the treatment, I eventually changed the name by adding the word "reprocessing."

I also discovered that other forms of side-to-side movement besides the eyes could be effective. Therapists could also use taps alternating from hand to hand or tones played from one ear to the other. Some scientists believe that all these strategies cause a constant refocusing of attention (back and forth) called an "orienting response" that links into the same brain functions that occur during REM sleep. Others believe that focusing attention on the trauma and the outside stimulation (eye movements, taps or tones) at the same time also disrupts "working memory." At this point, there is enough research for me to believe that both are true. So, if I had to do it over again, I'd simply call it "Reprocessing Therapy." But now Eye Movement Desensitization and Reprocessing—more commonly called EMDR—is known worldwide, so it's too late for a name change.

Why Does EMDR Work?

At this point, thousands of clinicians worldwide have successfully treated millions of people with EMDR therapy. It has evolved into a comprehensive form of psychotherapy with eight phases and many procedures and methods. Clinicians guide their clients by accessing past experiences that set the groundwork for current problems. Then together they process present situations that cause the disturbances, and incorporate new education, skills and perspectives into the memory networks that are necessary for future successes. The person receiving EMDR therapy not only addresses the obvious symptoms of a problem, but can also end up with a wide range of positive changes that affect all areas of life. That's because the memory networks at the basis of EMDR treatment have far-reaching associations. Changing the memories that form the way we see ourselves also changes the way we view others. Therefore, our relationships, job performance, what we are willing to do or are able to resist, all move in a positive direction.

Over the past ten years, the rapid treatment effects of EMDR have also provided neurobiological researchers with a "window into the brain." As a result, more than a dozen studies have used brain imaging (such as MRI) to document how EMDR treatment actually changes the brain. For instance, research has established that the memory control center of the brain (the hippocampus) shrinks in people with PTSD. For some time it was believed that since this was an organic change in the brain, the condition might be permanent. Happily, as brain scans have now shown, it is possible for the hippocampus to regrow. Although there has been limited research in this area, one study recently showed that 8 to 12 sessions of EMDR memory processing for people with PTSD were associated with an average 6% increase in the volume of the hippocampus. These effects were maintained 1 year later.

In fact, the first PTSD patient evaluated in this study was the son of a mother with bipolar disorder. He had had a variety of traumatic experiences in childhood and had a very shrunken hippocampus. After eight EMDR sessions, his hippocampus increased in size by about 11%. These types of results tell us that we need more research to find out not only how EMDR treatment works but also how an adult brain is able to change and grow. This "neuro-plasticity" is an event that scientists had long believed was impossible. Now that we know the adult brain can change, it opens up new possibilities for many conditions that were considered untreatable.

Even though EMDR has been proven effective, as with any form of psychotherapy—and most drugs—there are still open questions about *why* it works. Since it is a complex process, many elements are involved and research is ongoing. However, the use of eye movements in the therapy has intrigued many memory researchers. Therefore, an additional two dozen studies have explored the changes that occur with eye movements alone. They've shown that when people hold in mind disturbing memories or future fears, sets of eye movements result in less emotional distress, reduced vividness of disturbing images, shifts in thoughts and greater accuracy in memory. Of course, the eye movements alone are not enough for permanent changes. That's why they are embedded in the rest of the EMDR procedures. During EMDR therapy sessions, people remain awake and in full control of their faculties. However, one dominant theory is that the eye movements used in the therapy stimulate the same type of biological connections and beneficial processes created in REM sleep. Learning takes place as thoughts and information are consolidated and integrated with other memories during REM sleep. Research shows that if a person is taught a skill but is prevented from entering REM sleep that evening, the skill can be lost. During REM sleep, the brain allows the appropriate neural connections to make needed associations. The memory is processed and shifted to a more adaptive, usable form. That's why you can go to bed worried about something but wake up feeling better or with a solution. In a waking state you'd be aware of the insights that are occurring. However, those same beneficial processes are taking place while you are sleeping.

Unfortunately, as you know, some distressing memories persist. That's because the level of disturbance from some incidents is so high that the brain's information processing system becomes disrupted and can't take the memory to resolution on its own. This is obvious if you've ever awakened in the middle of a nightmare. The nightmare is simply your brain trying to process the information. The images reflect the emotions that are being reactivated. For instance, a woman who was molested as a child may have nightmares that a monster is chasing her. When that memory is dealt with during EMDR sessions, it's as if a veil peels back and the reason for the emotional disturbance becomes clear. The monster is the molester chasing her through her childhood home.

HOW MEMORIES ARE PROCESSED WITH EMDR

In EMDR therapy all the work is done within the treatment sessions. The client is not asked to describe the memory in detail or do homework. Instead, the clinician accesses the disturbing memory, jump-starts the brain's information processing system, guides the procedures and monitors the effects. As a result of EMDR processing, internal connections can be made rapidly during the session as indicated by positive changes in emotions, insights, new memories and a greater understanding of life issues. The dominant theory is that the original memory is accessed, connections changed and then stored with these new modifications in a neurobiological process called "reconsolidation."

We'll go into more detail about the different phases of the EMDR therapy in later chapters. But for now, we'll concentrate on how it directly "reprocesses" memories—how it taps directly into the unconscious and allows learning to take place. Research with trauma victims has found that EMDR is able to eliminate symptoms without the homework needed in other therapies. Also, since there is no need to speak in detail about the past disturbing memories, people who are ashamed of what happened to them, or what they did, do not have to talk about it. Significant changes can occur in a short period of time. We'll see all of this in the transcript of an EMDR session starting on page 34.

Before we begin, let me emphasize that we will be learning many EMDR techniques and procedures in this book that will assist you in both understanding and handling disturbing memories. However, during EMDR memory processing, very emotional material can arise internally. Therefore, it is vital that only a trained and licensed clinician conduct the treatment. This ensures that the information processing system remains active and the person is fully prepared and able to "keep one foot in the present." Trained clinicians know where to focus attention, what to do if the information processing system stops working again, and what to do if something unexpected emerges. As we will see, although starting with a major trauma—an earthquake experience where "Lynne" feared for her life and that of her child—there was much more going on below her consciousness.

Lynne lived in California and came to a research center for therapy because she had developed severe PTSD following an earthquake. She had actually been in two previous earthquakes, but this time the symptoms were bad enough that her life seemed unmanageable. One of the earlier earthquakes had taken place when she was in a college hypnosis class. Her professor had just put her under when the quake struck. However, it was years later that she became severely disturbed when she was home alone with her young son and another earthquake struck. I'll describe part of the session and then reproduce a section of the transcript that focused on the latest earthquake so you can see the brain's adaptive information processing in action.

Early in this EMDR session, the clinician and Lynne had already worked together to identify what needed to be targeted. She was prepared to allow the memory connections to be made automatically. The therapist then helped her to bring the memory to mind in a certain way. This included taking the measurements needed to monitor her progress. The image she chose as the worst part of the memory was trying to hide in the doorway with her son as the ground shook and objects flew off the shelves and crashed around them. Among other things, she also identified the negative thoughts she was having about the quake ("I'm powerless") and the emotions she felt when she thought of it. She had a high level of anxiety—8 on an 11-point (0–10) scale.

Then the clinician guided Lynne's eyes to move rapidly back and forth for about 30 seconds at a time. This is called a "set of eye movements." During each set, Lynne was simply asked to "Just notice whatever comes to mind, and let whatever happens, happen." Although she was completely conscious and aware during that time, new connections were made. Thoughts, emotions, sensations and other memories passed through her mind just as they might during REM sleep. At the end of each set, Lynne was told to "Let it go, and take a deep breath." After that, she was asked some version of "What came to mind?" Depending on her response, the clinician helped set the direction for her attention during the next set of eye movements. In this way, the clinician was able to take Lynne deeper into her stored, unprocessed memories and work them through to resolution.

During the first few sets of eye movements, Lynne noticed a variety of things, including connections having to do with "powerlessness" and lack of control. For instance, she recalled a tape she had listened to about people watching others get "smashed by trains." After more sets of eye movements, feelings of sadness and melancholy arose—this in contrast to the anxiety Lynne had reported earlier in the session. Anxiety can be a catchall for many emotions that are under the surface. After more sets of eye movements, she moved further back into the past. Laughing, she remembered running around her house with her brother when she was six. "I wanted to be a boy," she said, "and he told me if I ran around the house enough times, I would be a boy. I was disappointed because it didn't happen."

At this point we'll pick up with the actual transcript of the session so you can see how EMDR processes through the associated memory network, without Lynne having to give a lot of detail about what happens to her. When you see >>>>> it means that her eyes are being guided in a set of movements. It's during that time the associations and connections are made. Before each set, the clinician asks her to concentrate on some part of the memory and "Just notice." After each set, the clinician asks, "What's coming up now?" Then Lynne tells him a little bit about what came to mind, so that he can monitor her progress and redirect her if necessary. I'll just put in Lynne's responses so you can see how her mind moves from one memory or realization to another after each set. This shows the intricate connections of the memory networks in the brain. I'll also place some comments in brackets to help explain what is happening as we go along. Notice how each set reveals another aspect of the unconscious memory associations.

Lynne concentrates on the memory that emerged to consciousness of her brother telling her that if she ran around the house enough she would be a boy, while the clinician guides her in a set of eye movements:

>>>>>Lynne: Yeah, I was thinking about my sense of betrayal with my brother that he molested me, and how I really admired him [crying].

[Although on the surface, the first memory that emerged of her brother appeared to be funny, the deeper issue of betrayal and powerlessness is now revealed. Besides, even in the first instance, she had trusted her brother and he lied to her.]

>>>>>Lynne: Yeah [crying]. Something occurred to me like "Duh": How much—that it shook my sense of reality.

[Here we can see how unexpected and significant the different unconscious memory associations of the brain can be. The ground is literally shaking during an earthquake, and this is connected to a major event in childhood when Lynne's trust was betrayed. In both instances, what should have been a firm foundation was shaken.]

>>>>>Lynne: I was thinking about playing cards with my dad across the table from one another.

>>>>>Lynne: I was thinking about my dad taking me to buy a coat and buttoning the button of my coat, and pinching my nipple when I was like 11 and how absolutely stunned I was with that.

[Just as the first memory to emerge of her brother appeared to be harmless, this series of associations with her father also began innocently but then also left her feeling betrayed. Again, her father's actions give her the sense of reality being "shaken."]

>>>>>Lynne: What comes really clear—is getting sick when I was around the same age. Getting really sick with a pain in my side and nobody being able to figure out what it was and being rushed to the hospital. I really couldn't lower my leg and no one could decide what was wrong with me. I had a really bad pain in my side, and then they just decided that I had some kind of mental problem. I guess that was the only way that I could express it.

[Lynne knew she had a bad pain, but no one believed her, and they concluded that she couldn't trust her own perceptions. Once more there was no firm ground to stand upon.]

As you can see, unlike other forms of therapy, the associations to new memories and insights occur after each set of eye movements. The guided focus and stimulation allow Lynne's own information processing system to bring up spontaneously whatever is necessary to bring the memory to an adaptive resolution. The therapist keeps the information processing system dynamic and guides the process to make sure that the entire memory network is addressed. Now that you've seen how the spontaneous associations emerge, I'll describe the rest of the session and then pick up with the transcript again at the end.

As Lynne concentrated on the pain in her side during another set of eye movements, she realized what a chaotic and unsafe home she'd lived in. She remembered her mom and dad fighting and throwing things at one another while she was supposed to be asleep. She hid under the bed with her sister and tried to go to sleep but she was too afraid. The image of frightened children hiding under the bed echoes the starting image of her hiding in the doorway surrounded by the chaos of falling objects during the earthquake. It may also explain why it was this earthquake that gave Lynne PTSD even though she'd gone through two previous quakes. Cowering with her son with chaos surrounding them linked directly to her troubled childhood.

As Lynne continued processing her memories, she realized that she had wanted to protect her dad from her mother because "it just seemed really crazy." This thought brought her back to the most recent earthquake. She had jumped out of the shower, run to her son's room, grabbed him from the crib and run downstairs with him, trying to shield him. An interesting parallel emerged in her protecting both her son and her father. But this also brought her to the thought that she needed to safeguard her son when he was with his dad, who had been diagnosed with bipolar disorder and was on lithium. Lynne used to feel torn between letting her son be with his father and protecting him from his dad at the same time.

This shines a spotlight on the possible connections between our childhoods and later relationships. Lynne's original family was chaotic. Her stability was constantly shaken. She later married a man with bipolar disorder—a disorder that produces major mood swings. Her choice in men continued her feeling of being unsafe while once more placing her in the role of "protector."

We'll stop at this point and move to the end of the session about ten minutes later. She now realized that she wasn't "powerless." She had done what was necessary to protect both herself and her son. She felt she was capable of handling things in the future.

Clinician: Okay, so when you think of that original incident, standing in the doorway with Tim—how's that for you?

>>>>>Lynne: Well, what occurs to me is, yeah, that was an earthquake [laughing]. Yeah, that was an earthquake all right.

Recall that Lynne had been diagnosed with PTSD. At the beginning of the session, when she thought of the earthquake, she felt the same high level of anxiety and powerlessness that was present at the time of the original event. That is one of the symptoms of PTSD: The past feels present. However, by using EMDR procedures to access the memory and stimulate her information processing system, the appropriate neural connections were made and different associations automatically became conscious. She learned what was useful and regained her sense of control. What was useless (the negative emotions, thoughts and physical sensation) disappeared. Now the memory of the earthquake was stored in her brain appropriately. Since she no longer felt the fright of the earthquake, it had taken its place in the past. In fact, it evoked laughter. "Yeah, that was some earthquake all right!"

Not all PTSD can be treated so rapidly. There can be a variety of complicating factors that slow progress. A licensed clinician well trained in EMDR needs to carefully conduct the therapy. However, the research on EMDR shows that after the appropriate history taking and preparation, 84 to 100% of single traumas can be processed within about three 90-minute sessions. The more memories involved, the more time processing takes. But every memory does not have to be targeted since the other memories associated with the targeted one can also be positively affected.

Lynne's session is a good example of how processing occurs. It also shows the kinds of memories that contribute to emotional problems. For instance, the sadness Lynne felt during her childhood can also play a role in depression. And, of course, those childhood experiences can directly affect her choices in a life partner and how she responds in romantic relationships. In addition, the pain she had in her side that sent her to the hospital is an example of "somaticizing," where emotional pain shows up as physical pain.

This is more common than you may think. For instance, Jenny had been a gymnast and an avid tennis player but she began experiencing a pain in her shoulder, which stopped her from playing. During EMDR therapy, she realized that it started when she played with her father. He didn't like to lose. She had to suppress her own skills or she would beat him—and he couldn't tolerate that. After processing those memories, she never had trouble with her shoulder again. We'll look at these issues in depth in later chapters—including techniques on how to deal with them.

PERSONALITY AND PROCESSING

Lynne's unprocessed memories did more than just cause her PTSD. They affected her overall personality. For all of us, unprocessed memories are generally the basis of negative responses, attitudes and behaviors. Processed memories, on the other hand, are the basis of adaptive positive responses, attitudes and behaviors. When clinicians say "personality," we mean our usual ways of responding to people and events. In addition to genetic factors, each characteristic or personality trait is based on a group of memory networks that cause us to behave or feel in a certain way. These memory networks are created throughout our lives and reflect who we were, where we were, what was happening, when the network was created. That's why we can seem to be very different at work than we are at home. We can have different typical responses because we may have had a very chaotic home life when we were children, but we were very successful in school.

WHEN NETWORKS COLLIDE

Now that we've laid the groundwork for understanding how an individual brain makes connections, let's explore what can happen when two people with problems get together. *Barry entered therapy extremely distressed and nearly suicidal. His wife had just walked out on him, and he sounded like a broken man. "I tried so hard to be a good husband to her. How could she leave me?"*

Trudy returned, but their marriage was definitely in trouble. In trying to please her, Barry had completely lost himself. He was a sensitive man who rightly saw that his wife was in pain. She was wounded by her own childhood, and he wanted desperately to heal her. He tried to do things her way, rarely pushing to do what he wanted. Unfortunately, nothing worked. As she became angrier and more demanding, he became more passive and nonconfrontational. They were both being run by unconscious memories from childhood. Each was enacting patterns that made it worse for the other.

Trudy was the youngest of six children. By the time she was born, her mother had become depressed and withdrawn. Trudy's brothers and sisters bullied and abused her, but their mother did nothing to stop them. So for Trudy, Barry's passive attitude linked into her memories of her mother. She automatically felt insignificant and not worth protecting. She reacted to Barry by becoming angry and demanding, just as she had done as a child to try to get her mother to respond. Of course it wasn't "rational." Unlike her mother, Barry was trying to please Trudy. But once the emotions from childhood arise, they completely color our view of the present.

To identify the root of Barry's responses, I asked him to concentrate on the last time he and Trudy had had a fight. I asked what thoughts and feelings came up. "Powerless," he said. So I used a technique with him that we will explore in a later chapter, and his mind immediately went back to a time in childhood. He remembered listening to his parents arguing, and he felt overwhelmed and powerless. That happened a lot when he was a youngster, and it set the pattern for his marriage. His "old school" father was angry and critical of both Barry and his mother. He had beaten Barry into submission. In order to avoid the pain, Barry avoided confrontation and tried to please his dad. His passivity in the face of Trudy's anger was an automatic response. Unfortunately, it only incited her more as it linked into memory networks of her mother not standing up for her. For both of them, the other's actions triggered feelings of danger. As much as they loved each other, the past was present. It was killing their marriage.

None of us is immune from these types of associations. Our brains are wired to make them, and they happen all the time. Try this experiment. Choose a quiet spot and decide that for the next ten minutes all you will do is concentrate on your nostrils as you breathe naturally in and out. See how long you can do that before you find your mind has moved onto something else without your permission. It's very difficult to sustain this kind of concentration. That's why meditation classes take place all over the world. It's why Zen masters spend years practicing to hold focus on breath, chants or mantras. The brain automatically makes associations in relation to everything we do, think, feel. Our task is to recognize when we have thoughts, emotions or physical responses that are destructive, negative or harmful—and then do something about it.

WHO WE ARE

As you can see, while we are all the product of genetics, past experiences heavily influence most of our characteristics and our responses to the world. There is no doubt that how we grew up influences us. The experiences we encountered became encoded in our memory networks and are the basis of how we perceive the world as adults. And even the most supportive families can still leave children with unprocessed memories.

These kinds of problems can occur because childhood is a time when we're vulnerable. We're small in a land of giants. We don't have any power. So even in the best of childhoods, we may have experiences that are stored unprocessed with the emotions, physical sensations and beliefs that we had at the time. These experiences stay "hot" regardless of how much time has elapsed. In EMDR therapy the memories are identified and processed because they are often the foundation of current symptoms.

As we walk around the world now, a variety of things are happening in the present that may be linking into unprocessed memory networks. When that happens, instead of being able to deal with people and events as an adult, our childhood emotions and sensations arise and unconsciously influence our reactions. We don't get an image of the old event that says, "Oh, I'm acting this way because Mom forgot to pick me up at daycare." We just have the feelings connected with it. Once we identify and process these unconscious memories, the negative emotions and physical sensations no longer arise. Then we can be fully adult in the present and act appropriately.

I should also emphasize that not everything is based on early childhood. Many types of horrific experiences we can have as adults may cause symptoms of PTSD or other disorders. Sometimes it's an accumulation of those experiences that tips us over. But often there are childhood experiences that make us vulnerable, as in Lynne's case. Also, as we know, sometimes things that happen in adolescence can be very damaging. For example, Meg came into therapy because of extreme self-consciousness, shyness and lack of self-confidence. She always felt as if people were watching and judging her, even while she was simply standing in line at the grocery store. It turned out that Meg's problems stemmed from an experience in adolescence she had been hoping to enjoy. Her parents divorced when she was two and she did not see her father again until she was 13. She went to visit relatives in Florida and her dad came and got her for a couple of days. She was very excited and happy when he took her to the beach. Unfortunately, she had never been to the beach before and didn't know about sunscreen, so she became severely burned.

The next day, while at his house, she was supposed to help clean but couldn't because she was in so much pain as a result of the sunburn. Her father looked at her with contempt and said, "I can't believe you were so stupid as to not put sunscreen on." That visit was the last time she saw or heard from him. In retrieving the memory for processing, even though it was years later, it felt to Meg "like a kick in the gut." The shame that was part of that memory arose whenever anyone looked at her, causing her to feel insecure and self-conscious. Basically, it had poisoned her sense of who she was over the past 20 years.

Our brains are constantly making connections that are outside our awareness. Even during processing, only some of the connections come to consciousness. For instance, when I see an apple, it links into memory networks having to do with red, round, fruit, peel, stem, pie and all the other experiences I've had with apples. Whether I eat it or not is based on the feeling that arises internally. Am I hungry or not? If I had gotten sick from eating a rotten apple, I might never touch one again. The question is: Are we being guided appropriately by our memories, or are they pushing us to do things we shouldn't do—and preventing us from doing things we should? Eat it or not? Take drugs—or a deep breath? Stand up for myself or shrink away? Enjoy a success or worry about something happening to spoil it? Choose a relationship that's good for me or trouble? Be defined by "irrational" responses from unprocessed memories or mental health?

As we will see in the next few chapters, there are various ways to identify the unconscious memories that run us, and ways to deal with the reactions we have that come up to bother us. First, we have to recognize that some of our reactions are not based on the present reality, but are primarily caused by memories from the past. Obviously, sometimes anger, sorrow, fear or anxiety is appropriate—but other times they're not. Sometimes we're tricked by our reactions into thinking they are valid just because we are experiencing them. But just because we're afraid doesn't mean there is a tiger in the room. Roses are red—sometimes. And violets aren't blue—even if our minds say otherwise.

IS IT THE CLIMATE
OR THE WEATHER?

Although there are thousands of different ways to suffer, over the past 20 years it has become increasingly clear that what brings people into therapy generally involves one major theme: "I feel stuck." Very often they say, "I don't know why I keep doing these things." Or "Why can't I feel better about myself?" "I know I *should* think differently, but I don't." Or "I should be able to take action, but I can't." In other words, people are pushed into responding to the world in ways that are painful—prevented from doing or having the things they want. And then there are those who have tried to get help and say, "Therapy didn't work for me." What they don't recognize is that there are more than a hundred different kinds of therapy, so finding the right therapy and the right clinician can be the luck of the draw. But there are things to be learned from all the forms of therapy, and we'll explore some of those in this chapter.

WHAT'S IN IT FOR ME?

During my career I've given talks at hundreds of conferences worldwide. That's given me the opportunity to interact with thousands of people from many cultures in order to explore both our differences and similarities. What has been striking for me is that the same principles of brain, mind and body apply regardless of age, gender or location. In order to help you better understand how the concepts in this book relate to you, we'll try some experiments that I've used in almost every talk I've given. We've already discussed how unprocessed memories can affect people, since the disturbing physical sensations and emotions that are stored in the brain arise automatically. The body is a very important aspect of it, so let's try the first experiment. First, take a deep breath and release it slowly. Then close your eyes for a moment and notice how your body feels—and then open them to read the next lines. I hope you were not feeling disturbed in any way and have a sense of your body in neutral. Now take another deep breath and notice how your body feels if you close your eyes again and repeat some words. Open your eyes after repeating the word "No"—preferably out loud, or in your mind if you're not alone—for about ten seconds: No. No. No. No. No. No. No.

Just notice. For instance, did your shoulders, chest or stomach change in some way? Now take another deep breath, close your eyes again and notice what happens when you change the word to: Yes. Yes. Yes. Yes. Yes. Yes. Yes. Yes.

Did you notice a difference? For most of you the response changed, even though it's just one word. But the words have many associations to things in our lives, and there's an automatic physical response to what goes on in our minds. So what we'll be looking for in the next chapter is what stored experiences are pushing the automatic emotional and physical responses that may be keeping you stuck. Before we do, in this chapter we'll go over some additional groundwork, and learn some tools to help deal with any disturbance that might arise.

I should mention at this point that there are some of you who tried the experiment and got no reaction at all. It would be useful to see if there is anything to learn from an interaction I encountered during a workshop. During every certified EMDR training program, there are practice exercises so the clinicians who are learning the therapy also get the direct experience of what it feels like. The clinicians are broken up into small groups, giving each the opportunity to be in the position of a "client" while another is in the therapist role. Each "client" uses an actual disturbing memory from his or her life so that it can be a true learning experience. There is also a trained expert to supervise and monitor their progress. During one exercise, the supervisor observed a "client" starting to tear up and the clinician working with her said, "No, no, you don't have to do that here!"

Fortunately, the clinician was willing to be coached and the client processed through the memory without being asked to push down her emotions. As you may remember from the last chapter, in order for the spontaneous internal connections to be made, it's important to "Just notice whatever comes to mind and let whatever happens, happen." Then it was the clinician's turn to be a "client" and work on something from his own life. He said that he didn't have anything to work on except that the sound of his daughter's voice saying "Daddy" bothered him for some reason. So that was what was targeted. After a bit of processing, he remembered being about six years old on the porch of his house with his mother. She's telling him that his father had lost his job and was in another city looking for work. They are going to have to move from the house that he was born in. He begins crying and his mother starts patting him on the back and says, "Now, now, be my little man. Don't upset Mama!!" So, at six years old, he forces himself to stop crying and be a "man." That experience, and the sense that it was not all right to feel, became locked in place.

From that time on he pushed down his own emotions and became separated from any physical sensations of disturbance. Even though it was years later and he was a clinician—that experience still ran him, and that's how he related to his own clients. The bottom line is that it doesn't matter who you are; our physiologically stored memories are the basis of our current perceptions of the present. Unprocessed memories not only can intensify our sensations and emotional responses, they can also prevent us from feeling. So, the question to ask yourself, if you did not experience any difference between "No" and "Yes" in the exercise we did, is: Was the exercise not a good fit for me, or is this an example of generally not being in touch with my body and emotions? If it's the latter, there may be unprocessed memories involved. Because whether or not you're in touch with your body sensations or emotions, the unconscious connections of your memory system are still affecting your reactions in the present. Basically, the computer is still running, even if the monitor is off.

THE STICKING POINTS

Before we proceed, I need to be very clear about what is possible and what isn't. First of all, you can't eliminate unhappiness from your life completely. Things happen, things change. Emotions may momentarily come and go, as hunger waxes and wanes, as we lose, we win, we get good news and bad, Venus arises or the moon is in Bozo. The question is: How pervasive are the feelings and how long do they last? Meaning, is the sadness, anger, fear, anxiety, loneliness, shyness and so forth temporary and for a good and obvious reason, or is it the water I'm swimming in most of the time? Is it the weather or the climate? To figure that out, it helps to take a look at how often and where we find ourselves stuck.

Let's take Nancy, who came into therapy complaining of feeling anxious about flying. It had started when she took a small plane from one Caribbean island to another during an afternoon storm. Over time, she had become more fearful about upcoming flights. She finally decided to seek help because she had received a promotion that required her to visit multiple cities per month.

Nancy's problem could be understood and treated from a number of different approaches in psychotherapy. A psychodynamic therapist, for example, would encourage Nancy to explore her anxiety about flying in an effort to uncover her underlying fears and conflicts. She would be encouraged to describe what frightens her about flying, what her concerns are about the pilot, co-pilot, etc. Has she felt this way about caretakers in her past? Does she have problems with self-confidence and feelings of incompetency? Could her fear of flying be about a sense of insecurity in the world that she experienced in her childhood? Is her anxiety an expression of feeling unsafe in the world and is she angry with her parents for not protecting her?

Regardless of the underlying reasons, treatment would proceed as all psychodynamic therapy does by identifying the "conflicts" that Nancy has, interpreting them, and verbally working them through with the therapist to uncover the meaning of the fear in the context of a therapeutic relationship. "Working through" means to talk about the experience and reexperience it in the "transference" (transferring the feelings of childhood to the current relationship) with the therapist. At the same time, she will deepen her understanding of the present problem, her feelings about her parents and the therapist, and how her present experiences relate to the past. The exploration of these issues is conducted within a safe, caring therapy relationship to encourage the in-depth understanding.

Over time and numerous interactions, Nancy would eventually be able to better understand how she related to her parents, herself and the rest of the world. As she better understood her problems and developed insight regarding her own reactions, she would be better able to give up control in various circumstances. In this form of therapy, there is a recognition of the importance of past experiences, and an emphasis on reconnecting in the moment with the emotions and perspectives experienced in child- hood. The primary agent of change is the current relationship with the therapist within the context of "talk therapy." In addition to gaining insights and understanding, a psychodynamic therapist also might sug- gest some form of desensitization to help overcome the anxiety response.

If Nancy had been treated by a cognitive behaviorial therapist (CBT), the most recommended treatment for this type of anxiety would be a full day of therapy that includes a "behavioral experiment." In this case it would be an actual exposure to a real-life situation by taking a 45-minute flight together. Typically, starting from the therapist's office, the two of them would take a bus or train to the airport. Nancy would tell the thera- pist all the negative beliefs she has about every aspect of the trip, from travelling to the airport, waiting for the plane, boarding, all the way through to landing. After arriving on the first flight, they would immedi- ately check in again and take a plane back. The therapist's role is to pre- dict the circumstances where Nancy might think negative thoughts, coach her to think differently during the situation, and then compare what really happened to her fears. During the trip back from the airport, Nancy would be encouraged to summarize what she learned during the treatment and how these experiences can be built on to continue flying without the therapist's presence. In other forms of CBT, there would be multiple office sessions rehearsing the flight in imagination, often with daily homework.

In this form of therapy, while there is the recognition that something in the past caused the anxiety, the treatment focuses primarily on the present symptoms. The agents of change are the direct manipulation of behavior and beliefs. For instance, people who are fearful generally want to avoid the feared event or object, so the therapy involves facing the fear head-on. Since cognitive behavioral therapists believe that negative, irrational beliefs about what might happen are the reasons for the avoidance, the therapist designs a "behavioral experiment" or a real-life exposure to the object or circumstances to challenge these beliefs by demonstrating that the expected catastrophe—in this case an airplane crash—does not occur. In this way, the client is supposed to learn that the fear is unfounded and respond accordingly. In this form of treatment Nancy might be encouraged to take other airplane flights within the coming year and monitor her reactions with the techniques she had learned in order to prevent a relapse.

When Nancy took her problems to an EMDR therapist, the approach was very different. The focus is on the stored memories that are causing the fears. The therapist identifies the past experiences contributing to the problem, the current situations that are causing disturbance, and what is needed for the future. All of these will be addressed through processing. However, rather than talking about the disturbing experiences in detail, the treatment involves directly processing the stored memories, which allows the brain to store them with more adaptive thoughts and feelings. This form of processing simultaneously generates both insights and a "desensitization" of anxiety and fear.

So, guided by the "adaptive information processing" point of view, the therapist took a history that examined what had been going on in Nancy's life when she first developed her symptoms. Clearly, flying in a small plane in a storm can be frightening. But that happens to many people who do not develop persistent anxiety and fear about flying. Something else may have been going on. It also hadn't been her first flight. She'd flown without symptoms a number of times before she developed the fear. During the history-taking phase, Nancy and her therapist mapped out the first, worst and most recent flying experiences that were disturbing to her. It turns out that her symptoms started on a trip during her freshman year at college. Her parents had recently separated and subsequently divorced, a connection that she hadn't previously noticed, nor did she think was connected in any way. However, upon targeting the flight when she first felt the fear, her parents' separation came up as an association to that memory. She described how she felt responsible for her parents' decision and all the turmoil that went along with it at the time. She believed that if she hadn't left home to go away to college, they would have stayed together.

Basically, the buffeting of the storm during her Caribbean flight compounded her fear and anxiety at her home situation and became the basis of her anxiety about flying. But it didn't end there. Her feeling of responsibility for her parents' actions was not limited to their divorce. It's not unusual for children and adolescents to feel that they are to blame when their parents don't get along. That conclusion can get stored in their brain and cause problems later in life. But it was even more complex than that. It turned out that the excessive sense of responsibility was a lifelong theme in Nancy's life. Her father was an alcoholic, her mother suffered from depression, and Nancy had been put in the caretaker role.

After the memory processing procedures were completed, she no longer feared flying and went on the planned work flights without distress. However, at that point she had a choice. Did she want to stop therapy now that processing had eliminated her flying anxiety? Or did she want to address the larger issues, since it was now clear that she had an excessive sense of guilt and responsibility for her family—and everyone she dated. It explained many of the difficulties she had in her romantic relationships. There were a number of "care-taking" and "submissive" behaviors that didn't serve her, but she had just done them automatically without consciously realizing it. Over the next eight months she chose to continue EMDR therapy on these other areas where she was stuck, and the issues were resolved. That meant she was able to choose a good partner for herself and felt the joy of being an "equal" in her relationship. She felt free to receive love and nurturing instead of just giving.

Since we all walk around automatically responding to the world around us, it's important to begin noticing whether a disturbing reaction is appropriate. If not, is it excessive, is it there only in regard to a specific situation, or is it more far-reaching? For instance, I worked with a client who was pregnant and terrified of giving birth. Now there are many responses that are desirable in pregnancy, but being terrified is not one of them. So we tracked it back and it appeared to be based on the fact that she was the eldest of seven siblings. For her, giving birth was becoming her mother who had become prematurely old. We processed that and she very happily gave birth. It also affected the way she viewed herself, as she realized that for most of her life she had been overly concerned with her appearance, primping for hours before leaving the house for a party.

Whatever the inappropriate habitual negative emotions, beliefs and physical responses might be, they are generally caused by earlier unprocessed memories that are pushing them. The past is present. What we need to become aware of is whether the responses are appropriate. If not, do they occur in only one area of our lives, or are those unprocessed memories casting a wider net? Once again—is it the climate or the weather?

MAINTAINING BALANCE

Since we all have unprocessed memories that get triggered, we have all felt anxious, fearful, sad, angry or insecure at different times without really knowing why. Before we begin to explore some of those personal issues, it's important to have a way to get rid of disturbance if it arises. It gives us the balance we need to keep one foot in the present as we explore our past. Although we've all felt those negative feelings before, we can investigate most easily if we are not afraid of the emotions. The best way to accomplish that is to know we can get rid of them when we choose. Therefore, we'll learn some self-control techniques that we also use as part of the preparation phase during EMDR therapy.

A Safe or Calm Place

In adaptive information processing terms, what we're doing is increasing your access to positive memory networks. These are the networks that have within them the pleasurable experiences you have had in your life. For instance, the kinds of experiences where you felt calm and relaxed. That way, if you feel disturbed at any time and want to stop, there is immediate access to positive emotions. These are basically emotional state–changing techniques where we can shift our focus of attention and shift our state of mind at the same time—like counting to ten when you are angry can sometimes calm you down enough to deal with things. It doesn't change the reason you got angry or upset, but it gives you a breather between the cause and your automatic response. We all need ways of coming back into balance regardless of the reason we got upset.

So to begin, **we'll learn a "Safe Place" technique.** It involves guided imagery commonly used in hypnosis and meditation techniques. But with this technique you'll be totally awake and aware. It will give you a nice self-control procedure. Some people might find it easiest to record the instructions and follow them with their eyes closed. Leave that as an option if you need it. I'll also give some alternative choices in Appendix A.

We start with a positive image. What we're looking for is an image of a positive experience that you've had in the past. Maybe going to the beach makes you feel really good, or maybe the forest or a mountaintop holds nice memories for you. It should be a positive experience that is not connected to anything negative. Some clients will say, "Well, my safe place used to be in my closet with my teddy bear. Every time Mom and Dad argued I would go there." This is not a good place. Or "Oh, the beach is a really wonderful place except for the time I got raped there." That is not a good choice either. In some instances, people may feel most safe if they imagine themselves alongside a religious figure.

Identify a place that gives you a feeling of safety. Or if you prefer, it can be a feeling of calm. What we are looking for at this point is a memory that will help you retrieve a positive emotion that you can bring up and use to replace a feeling of disturbance. Please do not continue with the exercise if you cannot identify a place of safety or calm that is not connected to anything negative. Also, stop if negative feelings emerge. In those cases there are clearly unprocessed memories that will need the help of a therapist to address.

If you feel comfortable that you have a good memory connection that can bring up the feelings of safety or calm, we can do the exercise. Finish reading this paragraph first, and then try the first step. In a moment I'd like you to just close your eyes and do the following for a minute or so: **Bring up an image of that scene, and notice the colors and any other sense experiences that may go with it. Notice the feel of it, and notice the sensations that come up in your body—your chest, stomach, shoulders or face.** Notice if you're feeling nice, good, positive feelings, then open your eyes. Now try it. Did you find that bringing up an image and allowing yourself to be with it, noting the colors, noting what was in it, allowed those feelings to emerge? If the positive feelings came up, **now identify a single** word that would go with this feeling—such as "peaceful," which may describe the feeling, or "forest," which would describe the scene. That's a label for the experience. At the end of this paragraph, I'll ask you to **close your eyes again, and bring up the image, notice the pleasant feelings, and say the word in your mind.** Just notice the feelings as you allow yourself to merge into the scene while you repeat the word in your mind. Then after a moment or so, open your eyes. Now close your eyes and do it.

If those positive feelings came up, then do it again for another moment or so by closing your eyes, bringing up the image, and then bring back the word to pair with it. **Continue to do this for five times, spending about one minute each time.** This should help strengthen the connections. Try it now.

Breathing Shift Technique

Now let's try the exercise again, but this time notice the change in your breathing when you bring up the image and word. After you feel the positive emotions emerge, place your hand over the part of your stomach or chest where your breath begins. This is the breathing pattern you get when you are feeling safe or calm. That is also a useful technique because whenever you feel stressed, your breathing pattern will change. It will usually move higher up in your body. If you notice that happen, you can bring your breath back lower to that relaxed pattern. So close your eyes and try it now.

Testing the Effects

Now, if you've been able to comfortably go in and out of the memory, feeling the positive emotions and thinking the word, let's test it out. Read each paragraph in turn, and then follow the instructions. **Notice your body, and then bring up the image and word. Does the positive feeling come up with them?** Close your eyes to test it out, and then open them when you have the answer. Try it now.

If the positive feelings came up when you bring up the image and the word, here's the last step. **Try bringing up something recent that mildly disturbed you, and notice how your body changes. Then bring up the positive image and the word, and see if the good feeling comes back.** Try it now.

If it worked, then you can use this as a technique to improve how you feel when you are disturbed. Bringing up the image and word should access the Safe or Calm Place and will help you deal with those momentary problems that sometimes push us off balance. In order to make sure it keeps working, you should do the exercise on a daily basis when you are *not* upset. This will make it easier for it to help you shift from a state of disturbance to a state of safety or calm. Also try doing it with your Breathing Shift technique. **If you bring up something that bothers you mildly, close your eyes and notice your breathing pattern, then change your breathing back to the relaxed pattern by breathing from the area you previously identified**—lower down in your stomach or chest.

Adding Bilateral Stimulation

Once you have that safe or calm place, there is a way that can help to increase the positive feelings: by using bilateral stimulation with alternate tapping. However, it's important that you monitor your sensations and thoughts, and if they begin to change into something negative, stop and bring back your positive breathing pattern. Here are two kinds of stimulation you can use. One is just putting your hands on your thighs and tapping first one and then the other. When we concentrate on the safe or calm place we only tap slowly back and forth four to six times. That's about five seconds. We don't do long sets, and we don't do it very rapidly because the very rapid or long sets that we use in EMDR reprocessing can sometimes bring up unpleasant associations as new memories emerge.

Another way to do the stimulation is called the Butterfly Hug. It was developed in Mexico to work with groups of children following a hurricane. It has since been used all over the world to help increase the positive feelings of a "safe place." To do it, you cross your arms in front of you with your right hand on your left shoulder and your left hand on your right. Then you tap your hands alternately on each shoulder slowly four to six times. To try it, **bring up the image of the safe or calm place along with that positive word that you've connected with it and allow yourself to go into that state of safety or calm. And when you have that sense, tap alternately on your thighs or with the Butterfly Hug four to six times, then stop and take a breath and see how it feels.** Try it for one set. Then open your eyes.

If the positive state increases, once again just close your eyes, allow yourself to feel the feelings, and bring up the word. As you feel the positive sense arise, again alternately tap each side four to six times. This is a good way to reinforce and increase the power of the Safe or Calm Place so that you can use it to handle momentary disturbance. That can give you a sense of balance as you begin to explore some of your own unprocessed memories. Try it again. If the bilateral stimulation helps, then use it daily. If not, continue the image and word without it. Remember that you can also use your Breathing Shift technique to shift back into the positive feelings when you are disturbed. Use the Safe/Calm Place exercise every day when you are feeling good to make sure the positive emotions are reloaded and strong enough to help you get rid of disturbance when needed.

Cartoon Character Technique

Here is another useful tool that can help with negative self-talk. Sometimes we do something and our mind starts telling us how wrong we were to do it. What a big mistake we made, or we are. So you can try another experiment. Think of a cartoon character that has a funny voice, such as Donald Duck, Daffy Duck, Elmer Fudd or Popeye the Sailor. **Close your eyes and bring up that critical voice and notice how your body changes. Then make the voice in your head sound like the cartoon character and notice what happens.** Try it now. For most people, the disturbing feelings that go along with the voice disappear. These cartoons have such pleasant and funny memory associations that the negative can't last. Using these types of techniques shows that we can control many of our responses if we can just notice how distressing they are—and take the time to do something about them.

As I said before, these techniques don't get rid of the reasons for feeling upset, but they can get us back to a place of balance so we can deal with the current situation more appropriately. If we are dealing with chronic disturbing responses—negative emotions, thoughts, sensations and behaviors that come up often—these are generally traits that would best be handled by addressing the underlying causes. That can take some time, but knowing we have these techniques can help. We'll be learning more in the course of the book.

A COMMON SOURCE OF PAIN

During my hundreds of presentations worldwide, I've been amazed at how many similarities we share regardless of country or culture. For instance, I routinely ask the audience: "How many of you remember having been humiliated sometime in grade school?" Regardless of location or who is in the audience, easily 95% raise their hands. So, let's try an experiment to see if you have a similar kind of memory—and check on whether that experience is processed or not. If it's not processed, some disturbance may arise. If it does, you will generally be able to use one of the techniques we've learned to get rid of it. However, if you are already in therapy for a complex disorder, or feel that you might have one, please don't do this exercise. In that case, the personal exploration is best done with the guidance of a therapist, and this book should only be used for general information about the human condition and what makes people tick.

If you're comfortable trying the experiment, then close your eyes, notice how your body feels—then bring up that humiliation from grade school and observe what happens. Notice how your body feels and any thoughts that come up. Just notice it. Then imagine washing away the image with a high-pressure water hose or a large wet eraser, and open your eyes. This is another technique you can use to change negative mental images. Try it now.

If you feel any disturbance from the experience, then use your Breathing Shift technique or the Safe/Calm Place exercise to let it go. Now when you went into that experience, some of you found that your body kind of cringed—you felt the heat of the emotion that was there at the time, and maybe the thought that was there as well. We would say that your memory has not been appropriately processed because what came up for you along with the image were old negative or disturbing thoughts, emotions, physical sensations or beliefs that are part of what's locked into your memory system. Although you may have felt it in your stomach or your chest, its origin is actually in your brain. What you're experiencing is the result of the neural transmission from your brain to the glands and muscles of your body and then back again.

Remembering the disturbing experience triggers physical sensations that were associated with it.

Now examine what was going on in that memory that you accessed. Notice if it had to do with a teacher or coach, a group of friends or a bully. Did it happen in a classroom, at a game, at a dance? Whatever it is, just notice the different aspects of that memory and see if any tentacles of that experience are wrapped around your present. Meaning, do you currently have any issues with authority or certain types of people, issues with talking in public, issues about learning or performing, issues of discomfort in a group setting? Notice if you have any problems that might come from that earlier event. What aspects of that unprocessed memory may be responsible for restrictions you have in the present? You might want to jot them down for future use.

Now some of you went back to that earlier experience and the thought that came up was something like "Wow, she shouldn't have been teaching!" Or a chuckle with, "I was really something!" In other words, an adult expression came up with it, and your body didn't particularly change while thinking about it. We would say that experience has been fully processed and no longer contains the negative emotions, physical responses and beliefs that you had at the time. You can remember that you were upset back then, but you don't feel it now. The processed memory has been integrated into the rest of your memory networks and what you now have is an appropriate adult response to something that happened as a child. Consequently, there shouldn't be any dysfunctional characteristics in your present stemming from that incident because what's useless—the negative emotions, sensations and beliefs—has been let go.

Now why some yes and some no? It's basically the luck of the draw. Maybe a backfiring truck awakened you the night before it happened and you were so tired that the event just made a negative impression on you. Maybe you had earlier experiences in childhood that set a positive enough groundwork for you so you weren't affected. Maybe when it happened your friend came over and put an arm around you and said, "It's okay, it'll be all right." There is a moment, a window of opportunity right after the event, that allows a positive linkup to be made so it can be fully processed. Maybe it was genetics. There are respiratory and cardiac weaknesses, and there are different sensitivities to stressful situations that may overwhelm the processing system. But it doesn't really matter. It's a no-blame situation.

Regardless of why the memory is unprocessed, one thing to keep in mind is that there is no stigma attached to it. You didn't ask to have this disturbing experience negatively stored in your brain when you were a child. And you didn't ask for the negative aftereffects of whatever it is that happened. Just because the event doesn't meet the criteria of "horrendous" to an adult doesn't matter. If you think back to that childhood humiliation you will realize that it's a common event. Everyone has them, and yet for many of us it has had a lasting negative effect. That's because even though it may look small from an adult perspective, as a child it was not small. As a child it was terrible. Being humiliated in grade school can be the evolutionary equivalent of getting cut out of the herd, and right there you've got survival fear—exclusion potentially means death. Many childhood experiences are connected to that survival fear—not being loved, death. Not being wanted, death. Not being accepted, death. All of those survival fears automatically arise and can overwhelm the processing system. Basically, that's the way the negative experiences can get stored. So it doesn't matter whether it's something an adult would see as a trauma. If it has a negative impact in childhood, it can be the cause of present problems.

THE SNAKE IN THE GRASS

It's important to remember that while unprocessed memories exist and can be the basis of a number of negative responses and traits, that's not all we are. When we speak of processing, we are saying that the disturbing events are able to link up in our memory networks with adaptive/positive information. So, the humiliation in grade school links up with memories of other friends who were made fun of or ignored, and we realize that we don't think any worse of them. Or that teacher really shouldn't have been teaching compared to others we've known. Or those bullies are cruel and we don't want to be like them. We feel better about ourselves because we've had good experiences, good friends, and the memory of the humiliation links up with them. But when the disturbing event is too upsetting, it's stored in a way that doesn't let it link into anything more adaptive—even though the adaptive information exists in our brain.

For instance, if we think of the combat veterans from the Vietnam War who are still diving for cover, or who are still enraged, clearly there have also been positive experiences in their lives. They've read self-help books. They've been in group therapy. All of those things have happened and are also stored in their brains. They can function well in certain circumstances but not in others. They can be very loving to their families one moment, based on their positive memories, but enraged the next moment because something triggers their negative memories. The two memory networks haven't been able to link up. But it's never too late.

We'll explore those kinds of major events and symptoms in Chapter 6. But just to show what I mean, I'll give an example. Recently an 80-year-old woman urged her clinician to contact me. She was a child in Japan during WWII. She came in for therapy complaining of depression and anxiety. Her husband now had a significant hearing loss and his shouting and playing TV at high volume were triggering her. Needless to say she had major issues. Her mother abandoned the family when she was three years old. One day when she was in school, her father was conscripted by the Japanese army and she never saw him again. She lived through the bombings, and was raped. You can imagine all the hardships she endured. After a few weeks of treatment her life changed. She told her clinician, "I feel free for the first time in my life." Even at 80 years old, her brain was able to digest and store appropriately the unprocessed information that had been embedded for the past seven decades. Again, the message here is that it's never too late.

The bottom line is that nobody is immune from the possibility of unconscious unprocessed memories. You may look around and feel that others are doing much better than you. But that may just be on the surface. Sometimes a person can be extremely successful in the world because of positive, adaptive experiences, despite a terrible self-image caused by unprocessed events. For instance, Samuel was a 60-year-old priest and about to become the president of a prestigious charitable organization. Unfortunately, despite his ability to achieve, he had always struggled with low self-esteem, shame and anxiety. He wanted to free himself of these feelings because he knew they would be harmful to his new position.

During his EMDR history-taking, it became clear that his childhood memories and adult situations related to uncomfortable feelings and beliefs such as "I'm stupid," "I'm inadequate," "I'm not trustworthy," "I'm inferior." During his EMDR processing sessions, he addressed a number of childhood memories including being awkward at a restaurant, cowering on the baseball field, and trouble in Latin class. Then, the big one emerged. It was an early memory of his father raging, throwing food, threatening his mom, and being out of control. Samuel saw himself cowering by the heater. He couldn't help his mother and he felt completely inadequate.

That event set the groundwork for the later problems with his peers. The symptoms vanished after the emotions, physical sensations and beliefs associated with the memories transformed during EMDR processing. He arrived at the perspective of "I'm a worthwhile adult." Samuel was now able to accept the new position and perform his job without the feelings of inadequacy and anxiety he had previously felt. The positive experiences he'd had in his life were now clearly defining who he was, how he responded, and what he chose to do.

But sometimes, people can think their lives are fully on track and not have any idea how one of their unprocessed memories is running the show. They don't really know until it comes up to bite them. For instance, Paul was a European businessman in his early 40s when he came to therapy. For the first time in his life he was suffering from depression and anxiety (difficulty relaxing, concentrating and sleeping) that was affecting his productivity and closeness with his wife and children. Until this time he had felt life was good. He'd been successful in business, made a lot of money, and his family was well provided for. He basically had achieved all he'd set out to do. What was causing the depression and anxiety seemed obvious to him. He had recently lost nearly all his investments due to a combination of a downturn in the economy and a colleague's betrayal. Joseph, a man he had trusted, defaulted on loans they held jointly. He'd left the area, refusing to answer Paul's calls.

On the surface, Paul's depression certainly seemed to make sense. His investments had been accumulated over many years for his children's education and the couple's retirement. Until now, he had enjoyed a close and healthy relationship with his wife and children and they shared good friends. He was proud of his care for his family and his focus on their needs. But during the history-taking, some red flags emerged. Paul described a happy childhood until about age seven, when his father became alcohol-dependent, lost his job, and the family became poor. Paul was insistent during history-taking that his distress was related to his current financial situation and not due to childhood difficulties, which he believed he had managed to learn from and put behind him. But just to be sure, it's best to explore the possibilities. Is it the climate or the weather?

Paul and his therapist used a technique we'll learn in the next chapter and identified the "Touchstone Memories"—the earliest remembered events that may be causing current problems. One of Paul's Touchstone Memories included an experience when he was eight years old and was left behind at a family event. His negative belief was "I don't matter." When this memory was processed, *many* experiences in his life emerged in which he sought approval from others, particularly other men. During reprocessing, he realized his difficulties as an adolescent and young adult—low self-esteem, poor relationships with others, and drug abuse— were directly related to his early experiences with his alcoholic father. At that point he realized that his earlier experiences had affected him throughout his life, particularly in his relationship with the colleague who had betrayed him. He had wanted to help Joseph get started in the business. He now realized that he'd ignored Joseph's questionable trust-worthiness and work ethic. Basically, he had wanted to provide a mentor relationship that he had so longed to have when he was growing up.

Paul's father was mostly absent and was drunk when at home. He would push his wife around—and Paul couldn't speak up out of fear of his father's anger and physical aggression. Even though Paul was a good soccer player, his father missed all his games. He never felt he was good enough to get his father's approval. Basically his father was either angry with him or ignored him. So that set the groundwork for the "snake" that bit him when he tried to give a young colleague the support he'd never had. It's not an uncommon situation. We are all subject to reactions that researchers call the "halo effect." We see some trait in someone else that we feel good about and automatically we give that person all sorts of other good characteristics that he or she may not possess. For instance, we may relate to someone's sense of humor and think they also share our political views. Or we know someone is in a helping profession and believe they share our humanitarian goals. These are our automatic associations, and just like "Violets are blue," they can be totally off base.

Sometimes the associations are harmless. Other times, they stem from memories that blind us. Paul saw a young man who reminded him of his own childhood, and he wanted to help. The similarities also blinded him to all of Joseph's negative traits—making him think he deserved the help. Unfortunately, Joseph had been damaged by his own childhood. But unprocessed memories affect us in different ways—and unlike Paul, he couldn't be trusted. When Paul's memories of his father and of Joseph's betrayal were processed, it was like suddenly everything fell into place and he remembered all the things he had excused or ignored. These blinders caused by his unprocessed memories provide the same reason that many couples are drawn to each other in what turn out to be unhealthy relationships. We'll explore that more fully in Chapter 8.

The extreme depression Paul felt was also explained by his earlier experiences. His father's drinking caused the family to become impoverished. He felt his father had "lost his integrity" and "did not put the family first." So Paul became committed to doing it differently, providing financial security to his family and trying to be a good husband and father. But now his financial losses were especially devastating for him because he feared he would be unable to provide for his family—just like his father.

So, in trying to be different from his damaged parent, Paul had become a model citizen, accumulated wealth, and done his best to be available to his family. All wonderful traits. But hidden from view were the tentacles of the unprocessed memories that allowed him to trust someone who would betray him—and to feel completely devastated when his finances collapsed. However, after processing the memories of his father's actions—and his feelings of having betrayed his own family's trust—Paul's depression lifted. He realized that he had successfully accumulated wealth before and that he was talented enough to do it again. But now he could do it with blinders off.

Another thing to keep in mind is that identifying and eliminating the "snake in the grass" means it won't come up to bite later on. Of course, once we decide that we need help because we are feeling depressed, there are many ways to go. One way that people often opt for is medication. However, it might be useful to try psychotherapy first to see if medication is really needed. While antidepressants can certainly be useful in particular conditions, they may not be the best choice in other circumstances. In addition to side effects, there are studies showing that once the medication is stopped, the symptoms can return. For instance, a study published in *Journal of Clinical Psychiatry* found EMDR superior to Prozac for trauma symptoms and depression. After eight weeks, both treatments were discontinued and people in the group that had taken antidepressants began relapsing, while people in the EMDR group continued to get better. While antidepressants helped change the "brain state," it reverted back once the medication was stopped. EMDR therapy eliminated the cause of the depression. What we ultimately want is a change in the "climate," not just the "weather."

ON AUTOMATIC PILOT

As you can probably see by now, the cases in this book demonstrate how unconscious memories govern our reactions to the world around us. Like Samuel, Paul and Nancy, no matter how religious, wealthy or intelligent you are—no one is immune. Every association we make is based upon our memory networks—whether good or bad. The first step for any of us is to recognize what negative responses we have in the present. Then we can use some of the self-control techniques we've already learned, or others that are in future chapters, in order to deal with our responses. That means we need to monitor ourselves so we know when we are off balance.

Unfortunately, that isn't always easy because we are generally on automatic pilot. By that, I mean we walk through the world often just reacting to internal feelings, thoughts or sensations and to external situations. We may plan to do something, but our inner life takes over and we become distracted. To explore that, try another experiment: Make a decision that for the rest of the day you will only enter or leave a room by putting your left foot over the threshold. Write down your plan and put it by your bedside so it's the last thing you see tonight. Then this evening, before you go to sleep, see how many times you actually did it. If you are like most people, you'll forget more times than you remember. That's because the associations of our inner world become more immediate, more compelling than remembering to monitor our body and doing something differently.

A goal of this book is to recognize the unprocessed memories that may be running us so that we can be more aware of what is getting triggered and when. By using the self-control techniques, you can see how much you can accomplish on your own, and when you might need more help. Therefore, after a bit more preparation, in the next chapter we'll start to identify some of the memories that may be at the bottom of disturbing reactions you already recognize, or ones that may be waiting to bite under the right circumstances.

In the meantime, begin a daily use of the self-control techniques you've already learned. Remember to practice the Safe/Calm Place technique every day to strengthen it, so when you feel disturbed you can bring back the positive feelings. If you didn't find your mind moving into something negative, use the bilateral thigh tapping or Butterfly Hug to increase the positive emotions and sensations. You can also use the Breathing Shift technique to calm yourself when you're feeling stressed, and the Cartoon Character technique to deal with negative self-talk. Or use the Water Hose or Wet Eraser to help deal with nagging negative images. All these tools can help you to remember that you can be in control of your body and mind. As you explore your own unconscious processes, you'll find that understanding why things are happening can help even more.

CHAPTER

4

WHAT'S RUNNING
YOUR SHOW?

Most people seek therapy because there is a mystery to be solved. In more than 20 years as a practicing clinician, I've never heard someone come in asking my help because "My father didn't love me." People look for help because of something in the present. Basically, they are doing, feeling or thinking something they know is destructive, but they can't stop. Most people believe that even though they may have had an unfortunate childhood, it was years ago and it *should be* irrelevant. It's the *"shoulds"* that make it even worse, because *"I should be doing, feeling or thinking differently"* leaves people feeling even more like failures and increases whatever negative view they have of themselves.

ALL BOXED IN

One of the problems is that most people view the past as merely a "learning experience." They think, "Something happened, so I learned to feel or act in a certain way. But that was years ago. I'm older and more mature and I know it's not the right thing to be doing—so why won't it go away? There must be something wrong with me."

The thing to keep in mind is that there may be something wrong, but it doesn't have to define us. It means that there are certain unprocessed memories that are physiologically stored in our brains that contain the emotions and physical sensations that were there at the time of the event. Because these memories are unprocessed, they continue to generate negative thoughts and feelings whenever they're triggered. That's why you may have heard or seen some very successful friends suddenly begin to talk and act like children when they get on the phone with a family member. You may even see their facial expressions and posture change as they begin to feel powerless when talking with their parents or older siblings. The emotions, thoughts and physical sensations that arise can run the show unless we do something about it. *"I'm not good enough. I'm going to be hurt. I can't succeed."* These are the types of feelings that can emerge over and over again. In this chapter we will begin to explore what memories are boxing you into responses you don't want to have.

Let me emphasize that genetics and current situations needing to be dealt with can certainly be involved. The way our brains function because of a genetic load may make us more or less susceptible to the impact of different events. Our genes can also predispose us to developing different mental disorders if certain conditions are met. However, even in these cases a life experience is often needed to precipitate the symptoms, and other kinds of experiences can help combat them. We cannot change our genetics, but we can address our life experiences directly.

Working with millions of people, we have found in EMDR therapy that a primary cause of disturbing, out-of-control responses are the experiences that have been stored in the brain as unprocessed memories. Memories that have been processed naturally, or with therapist assistance, are transformed into learning experiences so that the disturbing emotions, beliefs and physical sensations are no longer held in our memory networks. Therefore, the ones that we're looking for, the ones that are *hot*, the ones that are negative, can be a single event, such as a major trauma that would form the basis for PTSD—or they can be more common events from childhood such as being bullied, being made fun of, falling off a bicycle, hearing your parents argue, finding out that a friend betrayed you, being rejected by some boyfriend, not being invited to a party—and the list goes on. Whatever it might be, those negative events, if they're stored and still hot, can have a negative effect on the present.

It's also important to remember that sometimes it's what *didn't* happen that is causing problems. For instance, being neglected at home, having a parent who was not available at a given time, most times, or during a thunderstorm can be a major hot spot. Children cry automatically because they are hard-wired to reach out and be responded to by a protector. If that doesn't happen, the experience can easily be locked into the brain as an unprocessed memory. It explains why many baby boomers sometimes feel a sense of despair that might not make sense. Think of how many babies were left crying alone and hungry in the dark because there were "rules" about how often they should be fed.

When we do EMDR therapy, the evaluation begins as soon as the person walks through the door. Basically, the therapist thinks of the problem as if it's a box with the lid screwed down, locking in the client. So, what do you do with it? You can hammer at the board or you can try to pry it open. But it's more useful to look for the screws that need to be turned in order to lift the lid. And that's what we're going to start looking for in this chapter. What are some of the specific memories at the base of your problems?

IS IT ALWAYS ABOUT CHILDHOOD?

Before we begin, I want to make it clear that we are all unique individuals, and not everything stems from childhood memories. While research shows that earlier events can cause us to become vulnerable to later problems, sometimes a recent situation can send us spinning because it's so horrendous. As an example, let me describe the situation with Tony, who was one of the first combat veterans I ever worked with. Tony had become very isolated since returning from Vietnam more than a decade before. He'd gone to live in the woods, and since I was offering free therapy, he decided to come even though, as he described it, "I figured, what the heck. I don't expect anything to work. But, you know, why not?"

Tony came in because he was constantly having panic attacks. Every time a plane flew overhead, he was ducking for cover. This severe level of reaction can occur with some patients having PTSD. It seemed to me from the intake conversation that there was a major control issue here. He was trying very hard to be in control, and when he felt control slip, then the panic would set in. So I suggested that we explore that feeling of lack of control by processing the memory that best represented it for him. He said, "Okay, sure, what the heck." He didn't expect anything to work anyway. He didn't want to talk about anything that went on in Vietnam, but he was willing to deal with the memory of his wife having had him arrested. She had gotten him drunk one night and got him to leave the trailer after having called the police. He got arrested for a DUI as he tried to drive away. This experience definitely represented his feeling of lack of control.

After processing that memory, and another one having to do with a failed sexual encounter, Tony said he couldn't be in control because "I'll probably fail the way I have with everything else." But now he was willing to talk about a memory from Vietnam. *He's a medic and his unit is out of plasma—so the CO sends him to another unit in order to get a new supply. He runs across the battlefield and picks up the plasma, starts running back, and a rocket goes off overhead and he gets knocked out. He wakes up with no idea how long he's been out, and both his arms are dislocated. So he bends down and picks up the bag of plasma in his teeth and goes running back to the unit. He drops the bag, turns around, and the CO comes running up and says, "Congratulations, you just killed two men"—because of how long he was gone.*

Together, we start processing this memory involving the CO and the authority issue—and how it linked into his father. After we processed the memory so that it was no longer disturbing, he now felt "I can be comfortably in control." When I checked back with him a month later, he reported that the panic attacks were gone. He said it took about three days to realize that when a plane was going overhead he was simply thinking, "Why don't they just get out of here?" instead of diving for cover. As generally happens, the changes after processing were automatic, without Tony even being aware of them initially. His panic reactions had been triggered because of the inappropriately stored unprocessed information. During processing, the memories had gone from "stuck" to a learning experience, and were now appropriately stored in his brain as the basis of his new healthy reactions.

The bottom line is that although Tony had issues with authority that initially stemmed from his relationship with his father, it was a horrendous war experience stored in his memory networks that was directly related to his panic attacks. He came to war as a medic and his desire was to help alleviate pain and suffering. Being told that he had killed his fellow soldiers despite doing everything in his power to help—while in a state of pain and exhaustion from his exertion after having been knocked unconscious with both arms dislocated—most likely would have caused problems for anyone. But the question is how long have the problems lasted? If they are not disappearing on their own over time, they need attention.

FINDING THE TOUCHSTONE MEMORIES

As we've previously discussed, most symptoms, negative characteristics, chronic disturbing emotions and beliefs are caused by the unprocessed memories that are currently stored in the brain. In order to make sense of a current experience, the perceptions (what is seen, heard, felt) have to link into our existing memory networks. When an unprocessed memory is triggered by similarities in the current situation, since the memory contains the distressing emotions, beliefs and sensations of an earlier time, we experience the world in a distorted way. Even though we may be 30, 40, 50, 60 years old or more, it's as if we are holding the hand of our young self, and it's telling us what to do.

In EMDR therapy, the earliest unprocessed memory that sets the groundwork for a particular problem is called a "Touchstone Memory." In this section you can begin to focus on some of your problem areas and the underlying memories associated with them. Therefore, since distressing childhood perceptions can come up when the unprocessed Touchstone Memory is triggered, before we begin our exploration we want to make sure that we can use the self-control techniques that we learned in the last chapter. Please make sure that you test them out. We'll use a 0–10 scale of emotional disturbance that's widely applied in clinical practice and research. It's called a Subjective Units of Distress, or SUD, scale. From now on, if I ask you to jot down the

SUD level, that's what it means—how bad it feels, from 0 (no distress) to 10 (extreme distress).

Take a moment now and bring up something that bothers you at a 4–5 (out of 10) SUD and then use your Breathing Shift technique or bring back your Safe/Calm Place. If the negative feelings go away, you can continue with the exercises in this chapter, because that indicates you will be able to use the techniques in order to deal with any disturbance that arises. In most cases, taking a few deep breaths and, if necessary, thinking of the positive image of your Safe or Calm Place will help clear your mind sufficiently. However, please remember to take into account the caution I've mentioned previously. If you are already in therapy for a complex disorder or feel that you might have one, please don't do the memory retrieval exercises. In that case, the personal exploration is best done with the guidance of a therapist, and this book should only be used for the more general information.

There are generally about 10 to 20 unprocessed memories that are responsible for most of the pain and suffering in most of our lives. These memories contain the emotions, perceptions and physical sensations that you experienced at the time of the original event. While the image of the event may not intrude on you currently, as it often would if you had PTSD, the negative self-talk you may experience is directly related to the perspective you had at the time of the negative experience. The knot in the stomach, tightness in the chest, the feelings of fear, shame or powerlessness are all directly related to the earlier event. The following two exercises can help you identify some of the earlier experiences that are the foundation of your problems.

We'll be exploring different aspects of life during each of the chapters. So, if you want to keep tabs on what you find, use a notebook to keep a record of your responses.

Starting with Recent Events

As with any form of therapy, EMDR begins with the client identifying the current circumstances that are disturbing. If the solution to the problem is for the person to gather information, or identify which steps to take to resolve a puzzling situation, then the distress will rapidly disappear. In many instances, in therapy sessions as in life, processing can occur naturally by reading or talking in order to make the appropriate connections. That's how all learning takes place—by making the necessary connections between memory networks.

However, when symptoms don't change in that way, more directed treatment is generally necessary. It's important to begin to recognize when an unprocessed memory is involved, since the way it is stored does not allow new learning to take place. So, as you think of the things that have recently disturbed you, are they ones that can be dealt with by getting more information, or by taking some specific action that you know will eliminate them? Or is the disturbing reaction you're having the most recent example of a long list of similar responses?

The reasons you give for your reaction may seem reasonable, such as "I always get extremely angry at work if someone is incompetent. After all, people should do their jobs right. I do!" But these situations arise all the time in life. As you look around your work environment, you see that other people don't get as angry as you do. Why is that? For one of my clients, it turned out to be because of his experiences serving during the Vietnam War; if someone was incompetent, it meant people would die. During EMDR processing he realized that "No one is dying. It's just a bunch of computers. It's nothing we can't reverse." For another client, the source turned out to be a classroom humiliation when a friend he'd counted on messed up their joint assignment.

If you identify something that bothered you recently, and it contains a disturbance that sets you off a lot, we'll look for the Touchstone Memory. Since your present perceptions are linking into a memory network, if it contains an unprocessed experience, those encoded earlier disturbing emotions and physical sensations can arise, and whatever you're feeling is going to distort your perception of the present event. In those cases, the current situation is *triggering* the old disturbance. To systematically keep tabs on what you find, label the first page of your notebook *Touchstone List*, and then draw a line down the center of the page. Label the first column "Recent Events" and the second column "Memories."

To begin, identify some situation that upset you recently or is still bothering you. It might be a situation where you know you were overreacting but feel emotional just the same. In some cases you might feel it was justified. In others, you imagined a problem might occur if you did or did not do something. On the SUD scale, where 0 is neutral and 10 is the most disturbing you can imagine, the recent upset should be at least a 6. On the first page of your notebook, under the heading "Recent Events," write a brief sentence that describes what happened. Just a few words so you remember what it is when you look back at it later.

Affect Scan

Now follow the instructions on the opposite page as you concentrate on the event that upset you. Make sure you use your Breathing Shift technique or Safe/Calm Place after you've completed it. Proceed step by step with the event, completing all ten steps. This technique is called an Affect Scan since it concentrates primarily on the emotion and physical sensation you are feeling. If this exercise doesn't work for you, don't be concerned

We'll be using other techniques to get to the memories as we go along.

Read steps 1–5 through once before you begin, and decide if you need to write down any of the answers to make it easier for you.

1. When you think of the incident, what is the most disturbing part?

2. What image in the memory represents the worst part of the event? For instance, the way the person looked, or what they said, or when the person walked away. If no image represents the incident, or you were anticipating a problem, just think of the worst part.

3. When you hold the image/incident in mind, what emotion comes up for you?

4. Where do you feel it in your body?

5. What negative thought goes along with it?

6. Now hold together the image and the negative thought, and feel the physical sensations in your body.

7. Focusing on the feelings let your mind scan back to your childhood and notice the earliest memory that pops up and comes to mind where you felt the same way.

8. On the SUD scale (0–10), how does the old memory feel now?

9. If you feel your body change for the worse, and/or the SUD level is 3 or higher, the memory has probably not been fully processed. If so, pick a few words to be your cue to identify the childhood memory (for instance, lost in a mall, slapped at camp, ignored by parents, alone in the basement, caught stealing in class).

10. Write down the memory opposite the recent event, including how old you were when it happened, in the "Memories" column along with the SUD score.

Returning to Neutral

Make sure that you use your Breathing Shift technique or Safe/Calm Place to return to neutral. If the image from childhood is too disturbing, you can also imagine it on top of paint in a can and just stir it up. The Paint Can technique can help to drive away the image, just like the Cartoon Character technique can help deal with negative self-talk. It's a good way to get a breather and give better access to the Safe/Calm Place.

If the exercise worked for you, and you identified an earlier memory that is still distressing, that unprocessed memory has likely set the groundwork for your reactions in the current situation. Knowing this can give you a better understanding of what's running you. In addition, knowing that your current reactions are being fed by the past can help give you the distance you need to deal with the negative emotions when they arise. When you realize you're being triggered, you can return to neutral by using some of the techniques we've already learned, and others we'll learn in future chapters.

The next section will help you understand your reactions even more. You'll then be better able to identify the source of your reactions whenever you find them to be a problem. Ultimately, the goal is to have more choice about how we feel, not be unconsciously driven by emotions beyond our control.

NEGATIVE COGNITIONS

Let's use this example to explain the next part of the process:

Jon was finding it difficult to function at work. He set his life goals low, expecting failure at every turn. He was prone to outbursts and rages both at home and at work. It was jeopardizing both his family and his career.

In EMDR therapy, we refer to negative cognitions—which are particular kinds of negative beliefs. Some forms of therapy would confront Jon's beliefs through questioning, written exercises and suggestions about different ways to look at them. In EMDR therapy, the negative beliefs are identified in order to access and activate the memories that need to be processed. These negative cognitions are a verbal expression of the emotions and thoughts that are a part of the unprocessed memories. In Jon's case, when he thought of the latest incident at work, his negative cognition was "I'm a failure."

Jon and his EMDR therapist used the Floatback technique, which we'll learn in this chapter, to identify the memory that was the source of his problem. His Touchstone Memory was of his father beating him for no apparent reason when he was four years old. The beatings continued until he left home at age 16. It turned out that he was being triggered when people used a tone or expression similar to what his father had used throughout his childhood. The tone some people were using at times at work and at home linked into his old memories and brought up the old feelings of inadequacy, anger and pain—so he lashed out in return. After processing the memory, his rages stopped. The tone no longer triggered him, and his feelings of being a failure also disappeared and were replaced by the positive belief "I can be a success."

Personal Exploration

To identify the negative cognitions that are contributing to your responses, begin by bringing to mind the disturbing recent event you started with earlier in this chapter. A negative cognition will match the incident—and the childhood event that set the groundwork for your negative reaction. You can come up with it on your own, or use the list of Negative Cognitions starting on page 84. The negative cognition isn't a description, so if you get triggered around coworkers who keep messing up, it wouldn't be "I'm overwhelmed" or "He's incompetent." It would generally be something like "I'm powerless," because it describes *how you feel about yourself* in the situation.

If we go back to early events in childhood, the same thing applies. So "Daddy was abusive" is not a negative cognition. It's possibly a description of fact, as it was in Jon's case. "Mother didn't love me" is also not necessarily a negative cognition. It may be a description of fact. But, if it's true, how does that make you feel about yourself? It may be "I'm not worthwhile" or you may feel "I am not lovable." Either of these two is a negative cognition. Likewise, if a rape victim comes in for treatment and says, "I *was* in danger," it's true and it's not an irrational cognition. But if the memory of the rape is unprocessed and she brings it to mind, the feelings that come up will include the sense of "I *am* in danger." This is an irrational belief because she's safe in the present. She's safe in the therapist's office. It was a correct assessment of the past, but the issue is how does it feel *now*? At the end of successful treatment, bringing up that rape should not bring up the feeling "I am not safe." But the irrational negative cognition verbalizes the feelings she is experiencing now, in the present, and these words are a symptom. They are an expression of the stored information. So we use the negative cognitions that we feel in the present to identify the unprocessed memories that are fueling them. If you identified the negative cognition that fits the recent event you wrote down in your notebook, just write it down underneath it in the same column. The same negative cognition should also match the memory in the next column.

So for instance, Jon's notebook entry about what happened to him when he was four years old would look like this:

RECENT EVENTS	MEMORIES
Yelling at Larry at work	4 yrs. old—Being beaten by father
I'm a failure.	(8 SUD)

IDENTIFYING THE NEGATIVE COGNITIONS

In the next exercise, you'll look at possible beliefs you may hold. While we may have many ways to verbalize our distress, they generally fall into three categories:

♦ Responsibility (I am or did something wrong)

♦ Lack of safety

♦ Lack of control/power

When I ask you to look over the list of cognitions on pages 84–85, you'll find a number of different sentences that verbalize the negative cognitions that fall into these three categories. For instance, under "Responsibility," there's a list of ways in which people may feel they are somehow defective: "I'm not lovable," "I'm not good enough," and so forth. Although we may know realistically that these negative cognitions are not true, they put in words the way we feel—and it's the feeling you have about yourself in different circumstances that ultimately controls your life.

For instance, think back and identify the first negative memory you had in your life. Since you were a child, it probably has to do with feeling powerless or not being good enough or being unsafe. Or it may be a mixture of all three. Take a look at that memory. Which of the categories does it fit the best? Being inadequate in some way? Not being safe? Or not being in control? It might be interesting to take a look and see if the same feelings fit some of the situations you have in the present when you overreact. The list below will take these feelings and put specific words to them under each of the three categories. Putting it into words will help you understand yourself better and identify the memories that are pushing the negative feelings.

As you read the list, remember that the negative cognitions describe the feelings we experience during our worst moments. In general, they began in childhood before we had any choice. Sometimes they began because others were cruel or uncaring. Or sometimes they began because of a complete misunderstanding. Like the little boy who stopped wearing shoes and became afraid of them. The therapist discovered that when his grandmother died, his parents told him that "her soul had gone up to heaven." So the little boy was afraid that the "sole" of his shoe would also make him disappear.

NEGATIVE COGNITIONS	POSITIVE COGNITIONS
Responsibility: Being Defective	
I don't deserve love.	I deserve love; I can have love.
I am a bad person.	I am a good (loving) person.
I am terrible.	I am fine as I am.
I am worthless (inadequate).	I am worthy; I am worthwhile.
I am shameful.	I am honorable.
I am not lovable; I'm unlovable.	I am lovable.
I am not good enough.	I am deserving (fine/OK).
I deserve only bad things.	I deserve good things.
I am permanently damaged.	I am (can be) healthy.
I am ugly (my body is hateful).	I am fine (attractive/lovable).
I do not deserve . . .	I can have (deserve) . . .
I am stupid (not smart enough).	I am intelligent (able to learn).
I am insignificant (unimportant).	I am significant (important).
I am a disappointment.	I am OK just the way I am.
I deserve to die.	I deserve to live.
I deserve to be miserable.	I deserve to be happy.
I am different (don't belong).	I am OK as I am.

NEGATIVE COGNITIONS	POSITIVE COGNITIONS
Lack of Safety/Vulnerability	
I cannot trust anyone.	I can choose whom to trust.
I am in danger.	It's over; I am safe now.
I am not safe.	I am safe now.
It's not OK (safe) to feel (show) my emotions.	I can safely feel (show) my emotions.
Lack of Control/Power	
I am not in control.	I am now in control.
I am powerless (helpless).	I now have choices.
I cannot get what I want.	I can get what I want.
I cannot stand up for myself.	I can make my needs known.
I cannot let it out.	I can choose to let it out.
I cannot trust myself.	I can (learn to) trust myself.
I am a failure (will fail).	I can succeed.
I cannot succeed.	I can succeed.
I have to be perfect.	I can be myself (make mistakes).
I can't handle it.	I can handle it.
I cannot trust anyone.	I can choose whom to trust.

Start by thinking of the last three things that bothered you recently—or that bothered you most this past year—particularly those where you feel you were overreacting. Write them down in the Recent Events column, skipping a couple of lines between each one. Then take a look at the list of Negative Cognitions. Hold the first incident in mind and see which negative cognition best fits it, and write it down under the event. If you have the feeling/belief that "It's my fault, I should have done something different"—ask yourself the question: What does this say about me? Meaning, does it make you think I am shameful/I am stupid/I am a bad person? Then choose the negative cognition that best fits and write it down under the recent event. If you can't find one that fits, just leave the space blank for now.

As you can see, I've also included a column of positive cognitions that counter the negative ones. That's how you would feel if you'd gotten the opposite message when you were growing up, or in any specific situation. Rather than feeling "I'm defective," you'd feel "I'm worthwhile." Again, this is a "no blame" situation. It just gives you an idea of future possibilities.

Putting our feelings into the words of the negative cognition gives us more information about our unconscious processes and the memories that run us. Rather than just having a "feeling," we can see that specific kinds of thoughts and beliefs go along with them. We don't have to beat ourselves up for having the negative cognition. It is just a symptom of the stored memories pushing the response. Let's see how many of the other recent situations that made you upset have the same emotion and negative cognition. Are they the same or different? After you've identified the negative cognition that goes with the first incident, then move on to each of the other incidents you've written in the Recent Events column and do the same. Write down a brief sentence that describes the event, and underneath it write one of the negative cognitions that best describes how you were feeling at the time. If you can't identify a negative cognition for one of the recent events, just leave it blank for now.

Now take a moment and explore what you found. Do all the events have the same negative cognition? Or are they different but in the same category of Responsibility, Safety or Control? Or are they in different categories?

IDENTIFYING THE MEMORIES

If you would like to find out where your negative reactions come from, we can try another exercise that we use in EMDR therapy called the Floatback technique. It adds another component onto the Affect Scan that can often help bring up additional memories. By using the negative cognitions to help access the memory, it can also give you a better idea of what's running your show. Remember that it's easier to do with a therapist's assistance, but this exercise opens the door to a personal exploration as long as you've found that your Safe/Calm Place and Breathing Shift technique are strong enough to close down the disturbance. If they are, then choose one of the recent incidents you identified, and move through the following directions step by step. Make sure to stop after you've identified the memory, and use your Breathing Shift technique or Safe/Calm Place in order to reset back to neutral. Then write down the Touchstone Memory in the Memories column.

Here's a brief example to show how it would look:

Part of Sandra's job as a corporate trainer was to speak before large audiences. But her anxiety was so bad that she tried to "prepare" herself with a couple of glasses of wine in order to perform. She identified the negative cognition "I'm not good enough." The Floatback technique brought up the memory of being in fourth grade. Her teacher singled out a few children to describe them to the teacher they would have the following year. She asked Sandra to stand up and told the next year's teacher, "She's a doozy."

RECENT EVENT	MEMORIES
Presenting in Houston	10 years old—Mrs. Alpert saying, "She's a doozy."
I'm not good enough.	(7 SUD)

Again, remember that there are no "shoulds." If nothing comes up, don't force it. If it doesn't happen easily for one recent incident, just try another one. For some people, a therapist's assistance will be necessary to guide the process. For others, there may be many memories that are all connected by the same emotion. So don't be concerned by the number. Jot down with key words the earliest one and the one that's most disturbing. Make sure to use your Breathing Shift technique and Safe/ Calm Place to return to neutral.

Floatback Technique

1. As you think of the negative cognition and the recent event, hold them both in mind. Where do you feel it in your body?

2. As you think of the recent incident and the negative cognition, notice the feelings in your body, and let your mind float back to childhood. What memory comes to mind when you felt that way? If something automatically comes to mind, then write it down in your Memory column along with your age and the SUD level.

3. Using cue words, list the earliest memories and the ones with the highest SUD level.

4. Place them in the Memory column opposite the recent event.

If you can't decide on an appropriate negative cognition for any of the events, then go back and use the Affect Scan technique we did earlier in this chapter. If you identify a Touchstone Memory, then look through the Negative Cognition list and see what fits best. When you hold that old memory in mind, how does it make you feel *now*? Sometimes it's easier to identify when you look at an old memory than when you're stuck in the reactions to current situations. Either way, once you identify one that feels right, you'll often find that the negative cognition will fit both the old memory and the present situation. Then you can write it down in the appropriate column.

Now take a couple of minutes to explore what you've found. As you look at the earlier experiences that you listed in the Memories column, do you see how they have been feeding your reactions? Can you see the tentacles of those experiences wrapping themselves around your present in any other ways? For instance, do you notice now that reactions at work and at home are fueled by the same feelings you had in childhood—or are there different events for each one?

NOW WHAT?

We'll do more exercises and explore more issues in the coming chapters, but for those of you who were able to identify memories, this is a good start. For those of you who weren't, it may become easier as we shed light on different aspects of your memory networks. And, again, please remember that some people need more help because of the characteristics that were embedded in childhood. There's no blame here, just information. Even if you haven't identified the memories, if you've identified the negative cognitions, that means you can begin to recognize when the feelings that go along with them are triggered in the present. We'll also do some other exercises that may work for you.

At some point, either alone or with a therapist's help, people will generally identify 10 to 20 memories that are causing problems in the present. These memories generally cause a physical reaction. That is, as you close your eyes and hold them in mind, you can feel your body react and/or will remember thoughts and feelings you had at the time. These memories are not fully processed. Each of these memories can directly affect your sense of well-being in the present. Some have helped forge your personality. Others can come up to bite whenever they are triggered.

While many memories may cause physical reactions, similar experiences are generally also connected within the same memory network. Major traumas can occur and remain unprocessed at any age. Other than those, the memories that are the earliest or most disturbing are the key to current problems. If these pivotal Touchstone Memories are processed, many others that are associated in the same network will automatically change as well. Once the memories are stored appropriately, the old disturbing emotions, thoughts and physical sensations no longer arise. Instead, positive emotions and thoughts that go along with the feelings of "I'm worthwhile," "I can succeed" and "I have choices" can arise automatically.

There are a variety of ways to handle your negative reactions in the present. One of them involves self-monitoring and using different self-control techniques to deal with disturbance as it arises. Now that the exercises have shown you how the early memories are connected to some of your current negative beliefs and reactions, you can begin to see the patterns that run you. That means you can also be more sensitized to your reactions and perhaps can say, "It's just my stuff"—instead of getting caught in the emotion. When you feel yourself get angry, scared, sad, insecure and so forth, you can use your Breathing Shift technique or Safe/Calm Place. If you get caught in negative self-talk, you can use the Cartoon Character technique. If you get an image in your head that keeps bothering you, you can use the Paint Can technique and stir it away or the Water Hose or Wet Eraser technique to wash it away. These and other techniques we'll continue learning in this book can help you move from one state of mind/emotion to another. You can make much better choices when you are coming from a state of safety or calm than you can from one of anger or insecurity.

TICES Log

Since one of the goals of EMDR therapy is to process the memories that are causing present problems, we ask clients to identify when there are situations that trigger their disturbance. A useful way to do that is with the daily use of a TICES Log, which you can begin to use to monitor your own reactions. Go to a new page in your notebook and draw vertical lines to make five columns. Put the letter T at the top of the first column, I at the top of the second, and so forth. You'll use the columns to fill in just a few words—bullets to describe your reactions to situations in the present that disturb you.

T—stands for Trigger. As we know, the current situation links into your memory network. If you are overreacting, it's generally because the situation is triggering an earlier unprocessed memory. So what happened? Was it a family argument, a look, a gesture, something said that left you feeling insulted or excluded, a problem coworker? Just list a couple of words so you remember what happened.

I—stands for Image. When you think of the event now, what image comes to mind? For most, it will be the worst part of the event. It's the part that really disturbs you, makes you flush with embarrassment, makes you angry, sad and so forth.

C—stands for Cognition. Choose the negative cognition from the list that best goes along with your feelings when you think of the event.

E—stands for Emotion. What emotion(s) are you feeling as you think of the event?

S—stands for Sensation and SUD. Where do you feel it in your body—and what SUD number does it have?

Once you've jotted down the responses, make sure to use your Safe/ Calm Place or Breathing Shift technique to return to neutral.

Remember, not all experiences are from childhood. Major traumas can have an impact at any age. For instance, Derek was an Iraq War vet who came in for therapy. Using the TICES Log allowed Derek and his therapist to identify the situations that bothered him and to search for any overreactions. For instance, after he returned home from the war, he discovered that he became upset whenever his son Parker cried. If Derek was holding him when that happened, he had to hand Parker over to his wife. The negative cognition was "I can't handle it." Here's how it looked in his TICES Log.

T	I	C	E	S
Parker crying	tears streaming down his face	I can't handle it	sadness/ shame	chest/ stomach 8 SUD

After Derek and his therapist reviewed his TICES Log, they used the Floatback technique. It revealed that the problem went back to an incident in the war. During a standoff, a woman was being held hostage. In the ensuing firefight the woman was killed, and her son had come out crying for his mother. The incident had understandably disturbed the whole platoon, even though there was nothing they could have done to prevent the battle. For Derek, the emotional disturbance he felt during the past war experience remained in an unprocessed memory that was being triggered by his child's distress in the present. After the memory was processed, Derek stopped overreacting to Parker's crying and was able to fully enjoy being with his son.

The bottom line is that whether it's an inability to perform at work or with family, friends or strangers on the street, an overreaction is generally caused by an unprocessed memory. If you use the TICES Log, you can choose to draw on the information in a number of ways.

1. You can use your answers to identify the memory that's pushing the overreaction by using the Floatback or Affect Scan. If you do that, write down the recent event, negative cognition and memory (with age and SUD) in the appropriate column of your *Touchstone List*. If it's a memory you already identified, then put a star next to it. That will help you recognize the ones that are especially powerful in running your show. I'll be showing you a variety of different ways you can organize the *Touchstone List* in later chapters.

2. You can keep tabs on how many times you respond negatively to different situations and notice if they seem to cluster around certain emotions and negative cognitions.

3. You can recognize that your responses aren't mysterious. They are not random. They are specific reactions to certain types of situations that trigger the unprocessed memories that cause the disturbing thoughts, emotions and physical responses.

You may feel afraid, sad, angry, insecure or powerless—but you now can also be aware of why you are responding that way. You are more than the feeling—you can observe the responses and do something about them. Using the TICES Log daily will give you the opportunity to review your day and clarify where you need to put your focus. Do you have occasional negative responses, or do they happen often? Do they happen with only one person in your life, or with many? Is it happening primarily when you are with family, on the job, with certain friends, acquaintances, strangers or alone?

Your TICES Log responses will allow you to become more aware of not only who you are, but also of what types of experiences and memories run you. That way you can prepare yourself before going into those kinds of situations. It will also help you to stay alert in order to use your self-control techniques to deal with your negative reactions and change to ones that are more adaptive. We'll learn more of these techniques as we go along.

Your experiences using these techniques will also help you determine whether you could benefit from a therapist's assistance. Some memories are simply more of a problem than others. Sometimes self-monitoring and determination are not enough. At times, the negative emotions can be too intense to step back from. If you continue to get triggered by the same things, then you can probably benefit from having the memories processed with a trained therapist. Guidelines for finding and choosing one are in Appendix B. It's the same as any other physical problem that needs attention. Your brain is no different from the rest of your body. You'd go to a physician to have your arm set if you broke it—then your natural healing process would take over. But without getting help to have the bones of your arm aligned first, it wouldn't work. The same is true of your memories and the information processing system of your brain.

In the coming chapters, we'll identify more of the memories that are running you. We'll also explore different problem areas that affect millions of people worldwide. If some of the descriptions ring a bell for you, it will help provide more information about what's running the show for you and the others in your life—loved, liked or otherwise.

THE HIDDEN LANDSCAPE

I n this chapter, we'll begin looking more in depth at the types of issues that most of us deal with. I'll give real-life examples in order to show the dynamics and undercurrents of why people develop a negative sense of "self." We'll also explore the reasons why many people can't seem to find a sense of satisfaction and well-being in life. The best place to start is at the beginning. Parental love is supposed to be the springboard for all living creatures. Babies are supposed to be nurtured and protected, as we are intrinsically wired for the survival of the species. It's through our parents' loving care that we learn the ways of the world and that we are valuable beings able to achieve our goals in life. It is through being loved that we learn to love in return. Except it doesn't always work out that way.

Here's a situation that is more common than you may think:

Lucille was pregnant with her first child. Although she was the youngest of three siblings, she was the first one to have a baby. Everyone in the family was excited and looking forward to the great event. But Lucille couldn't wait to get it over with. Unfortunately, just as she learned she was pregnant, her husband was transferred, forcing them to move far away from their friends and family. To make matters worse, she'd had a very difficult pregnancy—constantly nauseated and vomiting several times a day through most of the nine months. The delivery was no easier. She suffered through a long, painful labor that finally ended in an emergency caesarean section. After Lucille woke up she asked to see her baby. The nurses said she needed to wait until morning. But when they finally brought her infant daughter and placed her in Lucille's arms, she looked down and thought, "Something is wrong here. I don't feel anything."

Lucille wanted to love baby Amy, but couldn't. Although she wanted to do what was best for her daughter, she was not bonded to her. Instead, she just felt physically terrible and depressed. In fact, she was wracked with guilt about her lack of loving feelings toward her child. However, this was not Lucille's fault—or Amy's. The unprocessed pregnancy and delivery memories were stored in Lucille's brain, and those negative emotions and physical sensations were being continually triggered by Amy's presence.

Lucille tried antidepressants and counseling. They didn't change how she felt about her baby. So, although she fed and held Amy, gave her a bottle when she cried, and diapered her when she was wet, she had no feelings of love or nurturing. Instead, her emotions cycled between sadness, anxiety and anger. Lucille communicated her distress through the way she held and handled Amy. In turn, her daughter became fretful and colicky, which only made matters worse. It was the beginning of a set of problems that spring from lack of true nurturing and love. Neither Amy nor Lucille was at fault in the situation. Amy might grow up feeling unlovable, but she wasn't. She would have been loved if the situation had been different. Unfortunately, her mother's information processing system had become overwhelmed because of the experiences she'd had around the pregnancy and the birth. Lucille couldn't feel love for Amy, even though she desperately wanted to, because the unprocessed negative experiences were in the way.

Lucille's problems were resolved through EMDR therapy by processing her pregnancy memories, the current situations that disturbed her and allowing her to experience the good feelings that would have existed if the pregnancy and birth experiences had been different. After the EMDR therapy, in Lucille's words, Amy went from "being a chore to being the love of my life." This shift in Lucille saved Amy from a lifetime of potential grief and self-doubt. But others haven't been so fortunate. Ultimately, the parent/child relationship is one of the building blocks that helps define us all.

Once again I want to emphasize that sometimes there are genetic factors that cause or predispose us to respond to the world in a certain way. For instance, some children are born with a greater reactivity to stress in the environment. This can present a major challenge for parents. As I've said before, this book is not about blame—it's about understanding the human condition. As we explore the dynamics that influence the important early relationship between parents and children, it would be useful to see if you recognize any of these in your own family.

BONDING AND ATTACHMENT

People who grow up feeling unloved by their parents may be right. Thousands of women are in Lucille's situation without knowing what to do about it. For these women, while all their friends are joyously giving birth, they stand back feeling inadequate and empty. The reason for these reactions is generally the unprocessed experiences that involve physical or emotional separation during pregnancy, delivery or after the birth. This includes having a difficult pregnancy and/or delivery, forced separation during the hours after birth and a wide range of losses and emotional problems that could have started years before the birth. Some of the most common potential causes are listed below.

PHYSICAL SEPARATION

* Mother was separated from child at or after birth or in the following months.

* Mother had a very difficult delivery.

* Child was premature or sick at birth and/or was hospitalized in the intensive care nursery or incubator.

* Mother was anesthetized at the birth.

* Mother was very sick after the birth.

* Child was adopted.

* Other significant separation occurred.

EMOTIONAL SEPARATION

* Mother had emotional problems during pregnancy.

* Mother had emotional problems after the birth.

* Mother had a death in the family within two years of the birth.

♦ Mother had a miscarriage within two years of the birth.

♦ There were serious marital problems and/or mother and father were separated before or soon after the birth.

♦ Mother was addicted to drugs or alcohol at the birth.

♦ Mother moved before or soon after the birth.

♦ The couple experienced severe financial problems.

♦ This was an unwanted pregnancy.

♦ The child was a twin or triplet.

♦ Other event occurred that could have interfered with bonding.

The bottom line is that for those of us who have had the feeling "My mother (or father) didn't love me"—it might very well be true. But just as we explored in the previous chapter, without therapy the reasons might have been beyond anyone's control.

Lucille's lack of love for Amy was an automatic emotional and physical response based on all the things that had happened to her. Imagine the negative feelings involving the move to a new location that left her feeling homesick and lonely, the extreme nausea and vomiting during her pregnancy, the long and painful labor, major surgery (C-section) and her fatigue and feelings of depression after childbirth. It was all too much for her processing system to overcome without help. In fact, any one of these factors could have been sufficient to prevent emotional bonding.

Fathers can have the same types of difficulties based on their upbringing and the kinds of stress that occurred before, during and after their child's birth. It's also the reason that some children may grow up in a household feeling that their parents love their siblings but not them. It may be true, because of the differences in situations surrounding the birth. But if a child feels "Mama and Daddy don't love me," it generally goes along with the feeling that "There must be something wrong with me." It's not true, but it's encoded in the child's memory system nonetheless. While not all cases are as straightforward as Lucille's, as we'll see, there are many reasons why parents can't bond and connect—and consequently, why their children feel unwanted and unloved.

There are many factors that affect postpartum (postchildbirth) moods and the ability to bond, including traumatic birth, difficult partner or family relations, unresolved childhood trauma, unresolved pregnancy events and physiological changes in the mother's hormones. The experiences involving a C-section can also contribute to the problem. Given the increasing numbers of C-sections being performed, I should emphasize that while the operations may be necessary in many cases, it is good to be prepared to address the potential need for psychological, as well as physical, recovery.

For instance, Marilyn also had a long, difficult labor followed by a C-section. She was delirious afterward and couldn't really remember the details of the birth or what happened in the postoperative room. All she knew was that she was in tremendous pain, nauseated and weak. In the following weeks and months, she was afraid that all the trauma of the birth had affected her son Donny. She said, "I was freaked out being a new mom, and he cried after eating and was spitting up a lot. I was continuously wondering if I could have done something more for him. Was the eating problem caused by the trauma he experienced?"

The fear Marilyn felt is not unusual. Mothers who are unbonded often feel fear, unsure what to do or "nothing" when they first hold their babies. Because of her unprocessed memories, she felt distant from Donny. Marilyn second-guessed herself all the time. She always felt she was doing something wrong with him. She couldn't embrace her son with love. She was afraid she would hurt him—and Donny became more and more difficult to manage. After processing her memories in EMDR sessions, Marilyn was able to relax and enjoy her baby. She was able to feel and express her love, and Donny responded in kind. The irony is that until her memories were processed, Marilyn's inability to feel love was connected with a fear of hurting her son—and what was hurting him was her inability to feel love.

The effects on children who sense they are not loved can be devastating. As infants and toddlers, they may appear to be never satisfied—depressed, anxious, cranky.

When there is a continued lack of attachment, when the parents are not "attuned"—not sensitive and responsive to the child's needs—the result can be a lifelong trajectory of problems, including medical and psychological issues. Many of these children are deemed "troublemakers" in school and remain in this category later in life. Or there can be other negative responses based on what is called "insecure attachment styles." This helps explain how we've picked up a number of different characteristics that affect not only who we are, but also how we relate to others. In fact, these attachment styles can continue from one generation to the next, since the communication between parent and infant actually causes changes in the brain that shape how well we are able to deal with our emotions and how we view ourselves. These different attachment styles can explain characteristics you may recognize in yourself, family members or friends.

DIFFERENT WAVELENGTHS

When parents are attuned to their children, you can say they are on the same wavelength. It represents a "secure" attachment style. During the first years of life, these connections even assist the child's brain to fully develop in a way that helps them acquire the ability to remain calm during times of stress and relate well to others. The child cries and reaches for parents who respond with love and caring. The eye contact and interplay between parent and child is like a dance, with both moving in the same rhythm. This attuned interplay throughout childhood, where the emotional needs of the child are met, becomes the foundation for a secure sense of self and successful future relationships. Of course, as we have seen, there are a variety of ways a person's sense of well-being and happiness can be derailed. But happy home lives of this sort provide a good beginning.

Unfortunately, some parents are misattuned to their children. Psychologists estimate that this problem occurs about 35% of the time—and call these misattunements "insecure attachment styles." For instance, for various reasons springing from their own upbringing and later life experiences, some parents are uncomfortable with closeness and expressions of love and other strong emotions. When their children cry or reach out for them, these parents often automatically close off and pull away. In Joan's case, she reported seeing a video taken when she was about 10 years old that even at age 40, upset her greatly. Her mother was seated, and Joan came up to kiss her. Her mother moved sideways and backward repeatedly to avoid the kiss. Also, her mother never hugged her or used the words "I love you" since she said that being "too kissy, feely" was "cheap looking." One day, Joan overheard her mother say that she liked babies, but not children. They made too many demands.

So growing up, Joan learned not to ask for or seek comfort from her mother or father, who treated her the same way. She grew up feeling unlovable and kept her emotions to herself. Since she never expected anyone to meet her needs, there was no reason to express them. Psychologists would say that her parents had a "dismissive attachment" style—and that there was a good chance that Joan would parent her children in the same way. That's how things become transmitted from one generation to the next. Joan's parents raised her the way they had been raised. They cared for her physical needs, but not for her emotional ones. However, there was no malice—or even necessarily a lack of love. Their parenting styles were simply an automatic response that was no different from what they saw their own parents and siblings do with their children. It just seemed natural—the way things were meant to be.

Another insecure attachment style for parents is "preoccupied," where their own unsettling life experiences often intrude on them and they become overly anxious or angry. Sometimes they are responsive to their children, but when their own "stuff" is triggered, they're not attuned at all. Their children learn that they need to be very insistent to get their needs met. They can become anxious, demanding, clingy and overly dependent. Basically insecure, this carries on into their relationships later in life.

The remaining category is "disorganized attachment," where the parent's own memories of trauma and abuse cause them to pass the trauma on to their own children through frightening behaviors such as grimaces, angry outbursts, rough handling and beatings or through anxious behaviors such as flinching or fearful facial expressions. Their children find themselves in a "double-bind." The very person to whom they want to run for comfort is at the same time the source of their anxiety. As they reach elementary school age, disorganized children may become controlling and "punishing" of their parents—yelling, barking orders or throwing tantrums if they don't get their way. Other children with the same background may look frozen or depressed. They can internalize their anxiety and exhibit "perfect" behavior in an attempt to keep everyone happy. Basically, as with the other insecure attachment styles, the "sins" visited on the parents are passed down to the next generation.

However, once again it doesn't necessarily mean a lack of love. Parents will often say they are simply motivated by wanting to make sure their children grow up right. Nevertheless, their ways of parenting are often automatic responses stemming from their own upbringing triggered by their children's actions. For instance, Jenna's father, Harry, had been raised in a household with a "spare the rod, spoil the child" philosophy. Harry's father had used a horsewhip to make sure that all his children obeyed and grew up with a sense of responsibility. Harry in turn reacted to his children's misbehavior with loud roars, spankings and a belt.

Jenna, who was the oldest, got the brunt of it and grew up feeling like she always needed to be in control in order to keep from being hurt. But her younger sister, Clara, used to hide under the bed while Jenna was hit. She grew up anxious and afraid. Clara was so sure that she couldn't stand to be beaten that she tried to become invisible and withdrew—the quiet child who never gave any trouble. Later in life she became chronically depressed. For both Jenna and Clara, their paths in life were forged by a traumatized father whose "disorganized attachment" caused his abusive parenting style. It wasn't that he didn't love them. He had simply been molded by his own upbringing and unprocessed memories.

Happily, negative insecure attachment styles can be reversed through positive experiences with teachers, coaches, peers and therapy when needed. However, first it helps to recognize that the problems you observe in yourself or others may be based on these kinds of unprocessed experiences from childhood. Or perhaps you may be a parent who needs to take a look at your automatic reactions, since they can have lasting effects on your children. You may say, "Well, I was never beaten, and I don't beat my children." However, words can also cause long-term damage. For instance, Michael was described by his therapist as having one of the worst depressions she'd ever seen. He had very low self-esteem and practically no motivation in life. His parents never hit him. However, he remembered many times when his father gave him projects, such as cleaning up the yard, and then made him wither inside by grimacing in disgust and saying things like "Oh, that's all you could do?"

Many people feel depressed, or look at characteristics and responses that make them unhappy and think, "My parents were like this and I've been this way for as long as I can remember. It must be genetic." But that's not the only possible explanation. Remember, your parents' influence has been there from the beginning—and their parents influenced them as well. Even when there are genetic factors involved, the research indicates that experiences often make an important contribution. However, whatever the reason, it's not about assigning blame. It's about liberation. Whatever happened in childhood helped forge who you are today. As a child you had no control and no choice, but things are different as an adult. Once you identify your hot spots, you can use techniques to deal with them and see if you can locate any unprocessed memories that may be feeding them. To help in the exploration, we'll now add to the self-control techniques you've already learned and then move on to identify other memories that can be running your show.

EXPANDING THE SAFETY NET

If you were able to identify a Safe or Calm Place, then you already have a very useful technique to help get rid of a disturbance if it arises. It's important to use it daily when you aren't upset in order to make sure it stays powerful enough to work. If you keep using it only in disturbing situations, it can wear out. So if you didn't find your mind moving into negative associations, make sure to bring it up regularly and reinforce it with the Butterfly Hug or alternately slowly tapping one thigh and then the other.

Expanding the Safe Place Arsenal

An additional resource can be strengthening your access to good memories. So start by writing down in your notebook a sentence that describes a positive memory where you felt a sense of well-being, accomplishment or joy. It can either be a recent one or from childhood—whatever gives you the strongest positive feeling. What image represents the best moment? Close your eyes and allow yourself to feel it. What word best describes it? Then, as you did with the Safe Place, hold the image and word in mind and notice where you feel it in your body. Enjoy and let yourself savor the memory. Let it go and then repeat it a few times. See if you can bring back the good feelings with the image or word.

Seeing if you have a good, strong, positive memory will accomplish two things. One, the positive memory will provide a resource that you can bring back when you need it because you are troubled or upset. Two, it is a good way to check your memory base. If you are depressed, you may not be able to retrieve a good memory that brings you a pure sense of joy and well-being. Maybe you can't find a good memory, or you know it was a pleasant event when it happened, but now it comes up with a tinge of sadness. The reason is simple: Research tells us that our memory retrieval is affected by our emotional state. If we are depressed, we have trouble experiencing anything in the present or past as purely joyful. If you have been feeling depressed for a while, where nothing seems to give you joy, it would be useful for you to consider professional assistance. Some resources are listed in Appendix B. Also, it would be best not to do the exercises in the "Personal Exploration" section of this chapter. The next exercise may help you alleviate some negative feelings, and the stories may help you get a better understanding of what's bothering you—but it would probably be best not to delve too deeply into your memory networks on your own at this time. Maybe it's just a bad day for you and you can come back to the exercises at another time. But if your feeling of unhappiness is pretty much your usual state of mind, or alternates with other extremes, then read this chapter with the primary goal of understanding why these negative states of mind happen for you and for millions of other people. Then you can decide what to do about it.

Spiral Technique

This technique comes from the guided imagery tradition and is useful for dealing with upsetting emotions such as fear, anxiety or anger. If you practice it in the comfort of your home, you can quickly use it at any time. Read through the steps on page 108 about three times, or until you feel you can remember them. Then close your eyes and follow them in order. If you have trouble remembering them, read them slowly into a tape recorder and let your own voice lead you through the steps. Again, please remember that not every technique works for everyone. That's why we're learning a number of different ones in order to find those that work for you.

Identify something that bothers you at about a 3 level on a scale of 0–10.

1. Bring up an image that represents it for you.

2. As you think of the image that represents it, notice where you feel the disturbance in your body.

3. Now pretend that the feeling is "energy." If it was a spiral of energy, which direction is it moving in: clockwise or counterclockwise?

4. Now, with your mind, gently change the direction of the spiral in your body. For instance, if it was originally moving clockwise, gently change it to counterclockwise.

Notice what happens to the feelings in your body. For many people the feelings will begin to disappear as they change the direction of the spiral. If the feelings begin to disappear, then continue until you feel comfortable. If one direction didn't work, try the other direction and see if it lessens the disturbance. If the Spiral technique had an effect, practice on other situations in the comfort of your home until you have the steps memorized. This technique can assist you whenever you are distressed, and may be useful if we stumble onto an issue or memory that disturbs you. If it doesn't work, don't worry. You can use the Safe/Calm Place or the Breathing Shift or other techniques you learned in Chapters 3 and 4.

NEGATIVE COGNITIONS REVISITED

In the previous chapter you identified the negative cognitions that verbalized your feelings when you experienced some disturbing situations in the present. The Negative Cognition list is divided into three categories: Responsibility, Lack of Safety and Lack of Control/Power. You held the image of the event in mind and identified a negative cognition from any of the three categories that went along with the feelings that came up: I'm not lovable, I'm not good enough, I'll be abandoned, I'm in danger, I'm not powerful, I am a failure and so forth. Consider that a sampler, since the current situations you chose were those that came up most recently. Now it's time to do a more in-depth exploration as we look at different kinds of issues that affect us.

To begin with, we'll identify some of the negative cognitions from the first of the three categories—Responsibility—that may still be hidden from view. These negative beliefs can be triggered at any time—and can affect all areas of your life. So we'll go through the list methodically and seek out the ones that may catch you unaware. Look at the exercise as a treasure hunt. Then once you determine what's running your show, you can decide what to do about it. The negative cognitions aren't the cause of your problems. They are just the symptoms. As I've said before, the cause is generally the unprocessed memories that are pushing them.

We've already seen in this chapter how our parents' attachment styles have helped to mold who we are in the present. In addition, as you know from the exercise we tried earlier in the book, parents aren't always involved. Numerous kinds of humiliations in childhood and adolescence—being excluded, bullied, teased, insulted by a teacher—can have a terrible and long-lasting effect. Looking back, you know that children can be cruel, and some people shouldn't be teaching. But when the memories are unprocessed, it's the old emotions that run the show. All these kinds of experiences from parents, other authority figures and peers can cause problems that can be verbalized by negative cognitions in all three categories. However, the first category can have special significance and more nuances than the other two combined. So now we'll take a look at that category of negative cognitions and try to determine if there are any that might be affecting you in the present.

Responsibility—It's My Fault

This category means that the person feels they are to blame for whatever problems they might have. Somehow a feeling of being defective in some way became part of the psyche. There is the feeling of "I am something wrong" or "I did something wrong"—which also means "I'm defective" in some way. While many of these experiences can stem from our upbringing, they don't necessarily come from abusive or inattentive parents. For instance, 12-year-old Ethan was brought into therapy by his parents because he was extremely anxious, had panic attacks and was afraid of going to school. He had extremely low self-esteem, was hunched over as if he was trying to hide and was shy and self-conscious. His problems turned out to be largely caused by his overprotective parents who monitored every move he made. This was because Ethan had been born prematurely. Weighing only three pounds, he remained in the hospital for months on a respirator with cardiac and respiratory problems.

His parents' continued extreme concern for his well-being—they even became anxious if he ran—caused him to feel physically inferior and like a burden to his family. His feelings about himself also played out in class where his hunched posture and extreme shyness caused him to be teased and humiliated. All of these negative experiences with his peers made it worse until he became afraid to go to school. So the pivotal memories pushing Ethan's self-esteem issues involved both his parents and the cruelty of his peers. But the foundation of the problem originally stemmed from his parents' love and concern—not their indifference or malice. His parents' actions stemmed from their own unprocessed memories of the months they'd spent at the hospital and at home, afraid that their frail, premature baby would die.

Happily, Ethan entered into therapy at 12 years of age. But if he had come into therapy at 40 years old, complaining about unsatisfying relationships and insecurity, the basis would have been the same—his feelings of inadequacy rooted in his childhood. As an example of this, Elaine, a nurse in her early 60s, came for EMDR treatment in order to cope with her difficulty reading. In further exploring her complaints, it was clear that she had been suffering from depression and self-esteem issues all her life and had never understood why she had not been able to resolve her difficulties despite years of psychotherapy.

Elaine was aware that her mother's postpartum depression affected her. As a nurse who had seen thousands of women, she knew that when mothers experience postpartum depression, they are simply not able to provide the connection that their children need to thrive. She knew that all the times she reached out for a mother only to find an empty, flat space was not her fault. She also knew that she had been severely affected by the loss of her grandmother when she was six years old. She'd been Elaine's primary caregiver. But her awareness of the impact of these events hadn't helped to alleviate her years of serious depression.

In her history-taking, many early experiences were identified where the overall conclusion was that Elaine felt she was "not worthy." EMDR processing began with a memory of her sixth-grade teacher who told the class that Elaine and the other students who had scored in the 25th percentile would never go to college. This was a devastating experience that, 40-plus years later, even with her university degree, still caused Elaine to feel a strong emotional response. The memory clearly reflected her reading difficulty, as well as her belief that she was stupid and "not worthy"—unlike her smart and competent brother.

As the sixth-grade experience was processed, what came up in the memory network was the association to her grandmother's death and how she found out about it. She'd been taken to her grandmother's house. Since Nana wasn't around, Elaine went into the living room and got her Cinderella book to read while she waited. As she read, her aunt leaned over her shoulder and pointed to the word "dead" as a way of letting her know that her grandmother had died. It was a transformative moment in the processing when she realized that her unconscious association to the news of her grandmother's death with her Cinderella book was the beginning of her difficulty reading, particularly for pleasure. Over a few sessions, the target memory resolved completely with a 0 SUD, and her new positive belief of "I'm worthwhile" became solid and strong. Once again, it's important to remember that Elaine's aunt wasn't acting out of cruelty or any intention to hurt. But many experiences such as this can get locked into our brains as unprocessed memories. They shape our personalities and lead our lives in ways that don't serve us.

Although we may beat ourselves up for having negative emotions that we don't want or understand, most often they are simply part of the hidden landscape of our memory networks. No one is immune, as issues involving shame can affect a person regardless of how old, intelligent or skillful you are. For instance, Raphael struggled with feelings of inadequacy all his life. His mother had raised him. She was divorced and had a boyfriend in a neighboring town. Since Raphael's father was unavailable, she would work all day at home as a seamstress, cook dinner for her children and by 6 p.m. catch a train to the neighboring town where she spent the night with her boyfriend. She would take another train back home in the morning so she would be there to cook breakfast for her children. Unfortunately, Raphael had severe earaches as a child, and he was left feeling ashamed and "I'm not important" as he suffered alone, in pain, in the dark.

Now, when Raphael came into therapy he was in his 50s. If you had asked him whether it was right to leave young children alone at night, his answer would have been a resounding "NO." But regardless of how much information we have otherwise, the old unprocessed memories are stuck in their own network and haven't linked up with anything more adaptive. It's also the reason that combat veterans can listen with compassion to fellow soldiers speak of their wartime experiences, but beat themselves up as "failures" for having performed the same way in similar circumstances.

Likewise, consider the case of Marcia—a 69-year-old successful realtor who had the negative cognitions of "I'm not lovable, I'm not smart." Her father died when she was three, and her mother became physically, verbally and emotionally abusive. She would tell Marcia throughout her childhood: "If it weren't for you, my life would be better." Marcia never felt she was good enough. As an adult it was pretty obvious that her mother had multiple problems and was completely out of line. No one should treat a child that way. But knowing and feeling are two different things. The knowledge she had about what was appropriate was stored in a separate network from the experiences with her abusive mother. After processing her memories from childhood, Marcia now feels strong, with good self-esteem. Her past isn't different, but the way the memories are stored in her brain has shifted.

PERSONAL EXPLORATION

So, let's take another step toward identifying your old stuff. Using a word such as "insecurity" is like me asking you to picture the color green. I have no way of knowing what shade you're thinking about. Likewise, when you admit to yourself that you're "insecure," it is only part of the story. Different feelings arise depending on the circumstances, and different memories may be pushing them. Therefore, it helps to know what exactly is going on when you feel insecure at certain times in your life.

While in the previous chapter you identified the negative cognitions that are connected to a few recent events, they may be only the tip of the iceberg. The list of negative cognitions on the next page gives you an opportunity to get a better idea of your problem areas because the words themselves can link into memory networks with unprocessed memories. Since not only the thoughts but also the negative physical sensations from the original events are stored in your brain, they can help give you feedback in order to identify what's running you. We'll start by examining negative cognitions in the first category to see which are most hot for you. As you go through the list of negative cognitions in the next exercise, you'll be looking for negative feelings that go along with them.

Put a heading in your notebook that says "Responsibility." Then read through the steps below completely before you begin following the directions.

1. Look at the list of negative cognitions and then read the first belief—slowly and carefully. Notice how your body feels as you read the words.

2. As you read the negative belief, does it give you an uncomfortable feeling in your body or cause your breathing to change (quicken, shorten, catch)? If it does, then write it down in your notebook under the heading "Responsibility."

3. Take a few deep breaths to let go of the negative feelings. Wait enough time for your body to return to neutral before you continue. If you need additional help, use the Safe Place or Breathing Shift techniques you learned in the previous chapters.

4. Continue down the list with each one—slowly and carefully—as you notice whether or not you have a body response.

5. Write down each cognition that causes a response—taking a few deep breaths between each one.

Don't judge what *should be* happening. Just notice. As I mentioned in an earlier chapter, some people are not sensitive to body changes. If that's the case, don't worry if the exercise doesn't work for you.

Now begin with the list below:

Responsibility: Being Defective

I don't deserve love.

I am a bad person.

I am terrible.

I am worthless (inadequate).

I am shameful.

I am not lovable.

I am not good enough.

I deserve only bad things.

I am permanently damaged.

I am ugly (my body is hateful).

I do not deserve . . .

I am stupid (not smart enough).

I am insignificant (unimportant).

I am a disappointment.

I deserve to die.

I deserve to be miserable.

I am different (don't belong).

Now try these statements below. If they seem to fit, ask yourself, "What does this say about me?" For instance, I am shameful/I am stupid/I am worthless.

I should have done something.

I did something wrong.

I should have known better.

Exploring the Landscape

What negative cognitions resonate for you? You may have found a number of negative cognitions in this category, or none at all. Remember that the words of each belief simply verbalize the emotion and perspective that is stored in your unprocessed memory networks. Take a look at some of the things that have most upset you in the past few years. Do these words match the feelings you were having? Do you see the kinds of situations that trigger your negative reactions?

If you do, then you can prepare yourself in advance by pumping up the self-control techniques before going into the situations—such as the Safe Place or other positive memory connections you identified earlier in this chapter. That way, if you do get triggered, you can use the Breathing Shift technique, Safe/Calm Place or positive memory to handle the disturbance. Afterward, if there are still negative feelings, you can use the Paint Can, Cartoon Character or Spiral techniques to help get rid of the residue. Basically, you get to see that your negative feelings are just predictable responses as the situations in the present interact with your memory networks, and the emotions and physical sensations arise. Rather than getting sucked in, you may have enough of a breathing space to shift gears.

Identifying the Memories

If you like, you can now identify more of the Touchstone Memories that are pushing these negative feelings. The cognitions that resonate for you are the ones that most correspond to feelings you may commonly have of shame, fear, anger, sadness or helplessness. Remember that your situation is no different from the people you've read about in this chapter. There is nothing shameful about having unprocessed memories. We all have them. It was all the luck of the draw based on a combination of genetics, upbringing and a number of other factors over which we had no control. It's a no-blame situation.

So, for each of the negative cognitions you wrote down, you may be able to use the Floatback technique to identify the memory by proceeding through the following directions, step by step. Some may need a therapist's assistance. Remember, Elaine's memory of being told about her grandmother's death while reading a book only came up during her processing. Regardless of whether or not one memory comes up for each negative cognition, I suggest not trying more than a couple of them at a time. Give yourself a breather and spread it out over a few days. Also, make sure to stop after you've completed the exercise for each belief, and use your Breathing Shift technique or Safe/Calm Place in order to reset back to neutral. If the Floatback technique doesn't work for you now, step away from it and come back to it at a later time. Don't try to force it. Just let whatever happens, happen.

Read the steps through until you memorize them, and then go through them with the first negative cognition on your personal list.

1. As you think of the negative cognition, when have you felt that recently? What incident occurred? Hold that in mind. If no recent event comes to mind, just concentrate on the belief. Where do you feel it in your body?

2. As you think of the recent incident (if you have one) and the negative belief—for instance, think the words "I'm different"— notice the feeling, and let your mind float back to childhood. What memory appears when you felt that way? Something may automatically come to mind. Write the recent event, negative cognition and memory in the appropriate column of your list.

3. If you locate a memory, on a SUD scale of 0 to 10, how does it feel
    now? Write it down along with the age you were when it occurred.

If nothing comes to mind, specifically hold the belief and body sensation in mind and think of your parents. If you find an early memory that
pops up, then write it down. If not, then see if one comes up as you think
individually of your siblings and other family members. If not, then scan
for a memory of your teachers, your peers (school/camp/neighborhood),
or other significant figures in your life. Hold the negative belief in mind
as you think of them separately and see if a memory emerges. Just jot
down with key words any early memory that resonates with that negative cognition. Make sure to use your Breathing Shift technique and
Safe/Calm Place to return to neutral. You can also try a Belly Breath,
which can help to lower your disturbance. Inhale slowly and deeply for
a slow count of five. Feel your belly expand as it fills with air. Then
slowly let it out. Concentrate on your belly expanding and contracting as
you inhale and then release your breath. Repeat about a dozen times to
help return to a state of calm.

SELF-CARE

If you've identified any personal negative cognitions and the memory
pushing them, take the opportunity to feel some compassion for what
you went through as a child. That doesn't mean self-pity. It means having the same feeling of understanding and tenderness you might have for
any hurting child. Just as the people in this book who have shared their
stories, each of us is a product of how our brain works—and the memories that were stored in it without our consent or control. See if you can
also feel compassion for yourself as you are right now.

We'll continue with other personal exercises in later chapters and when we're done, you'll have a better idea of what's running your show. That includes why you may have chronic feelings of anxiety, sadness or anger. If your negative responses are occasional, you will also have a good idea of the kinds of situations that will kick up your disturbing feelings. You can then prepare yourself in advance with the Safe/Calm Place exercise when you know you'll be encountering those circumstances, or use it afterward if the negative emotions and sensations arise. You can also use the Spiral and other techniques to get rid of distress. There is a glossary and self-help techniques in Appendix A as a reminder and quick review.

We'll be learning additional techniques as we go along to help you deal with your automatic responses—and you can do quite a bit by monitoring your reactions and using these tools. The question in the long run is: Does this do enough to satisfy you? If not, you might consider processing the touchstone memories you identify with a therapist. A goal of EMDR therapy is to "digest" the old, stuck experiences, so those physical sensations and emotions are no longer pushing you in directions you don't want to go. Most important, that means the negative feelings and cognitions are transformed to positive ones—and you are freed to experience life with a new sense of empowerment and well-being. As you've already begun to observe, these memories can underlie problems and stifle personal happiness in extremely widespread and unexpected ways. Now that you realize it, you can make your own choices about reshaping that previously hidden landscape.

I WOULD IF I COULD,
BUT I CAN'T

J ust like love, sorrow and anger—anxiety and fear are important and useful emotions. They alert us to potentially difficult or dangerous situations that may need to be addressed. They provide warning signals to guide our next moves—such as investigating whether the danger is real, and what we need to do to deal with it. We all have these feelings occasionally. They are natural responses to certain situations and people that we encounter, and they serve us well—unless they're misplaced. Unfortunately, in many cases anxiety and fear increase out of proportion to reality and become connected to things, situations and activities that don't really make sense. Yes, a snarling, lunging Rottweiler is a good reason to feel fear and back off. A poodle on a leash mildly walking along the street is not. But for a person with a dog phobia, just seeing a picture of a dog can cause a fear reaction.

There are millions of people suffering from inappropriate fear, but not all seek therapy. Although they are not as happy as they could be, fear generally goes along with the natural reaction to stay away from things and situations that bother us. If we can avoid them successfully, we often plan our lives accordingly. Therefore, even though surveys in the US have shown that fear of public speaking comes in first, even before fear of death, most people just avoid public speaking and don't think about it. People typically only seek therapy if their job suddenly demands that they do it—or they realize that the fear is holding them back in some other way, such as preventing them from promoting a cause they believe in. But for others, it's impossible to avoid some situations that are causing fear and anxiety. This chapter will explore the intricate connections that can cause these disturbances.

Let's start with the case of 14-year-old James, who suffered from anxiety whenever he had to go to bed. He was afraid of being killed in his sleep by someone sneaking into his room while he was alone. It became so bad that he had to decide whether to sleep with his back toward or away from the door. He decided that it was better to sleep facing away from it, because then he'd just be killed by someone from behind without knowing, instead of having to see the person coming toward him and being helpless to do anything.

As it is for many people, James couldn't identify the cause of his fear, but it had been going on for years, getting progressively worse. So his therapist asked him to remember the feelings he'd had the night before in order to access his memory network. As James concentrated on the image and fear of going to sleep alone in his room, the processing began. What emerged was that six years earlier, when he was eight years old, his parents had gone on a trip and left him with his grandmother. It was during the time that the newspapers and TV were filled with stories of the Night Stalker murders in California. People were worried about where he might strike next and there was a pervasive sense of alarm. James' brain had linked his parents' absence with the murders. After that, when he went to sleep alone in his room, the sense of danger and anxiety emerged. His symptoms disappeared after the memory was processed.

Happily, James' parents had brought him in for therapy when he was 14 years old. Unfortunately, millions of other people continue to suffer needlessly, feeling anxious and fearful about a wide variety of things. Sometimes the feelings are linked to specific circumstances, but sometimes they seem to be ever present. Regardless of the cause, it would help to remember that there is generally something stored in the memory network that started it—even if you haven't been able to identify what it is.

THEM AGAIN?

Not surprisingly, when people have a pervasive feeling of anxiety and fear, it can stem from feelings connected to the insecure attachment styles we discussed in the previous chapter. Do I mean that we're back to the parents again? Yes. Unfortunately, feelings of lack of safety and security can be based on the fact that we didn't feel sufficiently valued and protected as children. We were left feeling that we weren't good enough, and worried that other people would negatively judge us.

Sometimes those feelings are compounded by additional problems. For instance, Laura was hospitalized for the first eight months of her life for surgeries to address a disfigurement at birth. Although the surgeries were successful, the eight-month removal from her home took its toll. She never felt close to her parents. Her anxiety made her come in for therapy because she couldn't allow herself to be close to people. She even dreaded getting hugs from friends. Although she had her own business and was very successful, her negative beliefs were "It's not safe to be close to people. They don't really care." There were two childhood memories that needed to be processed. One was her having to sit on her father's lap for a photographer. She felt that Dad was "pretending" to like her. The second was a similar memory of her mother "pretending" to care. She was able to process these memories and then process current triggers with friends. She felt she could now accept her friends' hugs. She could then strongly feel the positive beliefs: "It's safe to be close. They really do care."

Now, whether or not her parents really loved her but had difficulty showing it, or the forced separation from Laura as a baby disrupted their ability to bond, makes very little difference. Children take on the blame for their parents' missteps. They also take on the feelings that are being generated in the household. If a parent is preoccupied with an over-whelming situation, for whatever reasons, children simply may not get their needs met. For instance, Ava probably had "good" parents. But unfortunately, throughout Ava's childhood her mother was battling can-cer, and it had affected her sense of security. Then when Ava was 16 she lost her mother to the disease.

Growing up in this way can cause pervasive feelings of anxiety and a negative sense of self. However, people might not recognize this low-grade tension in their lives because they've never known anything differ-ent. It generally takes some escalation of emotional pain in order to recognize that help is needed. Ava came in for therapy because after a recent breakup she recognized that she had become dependent upon men and continued to get involved in unhealthy relationships. Her identified negative cognition was "It's not safe to be alone"—and it became clear that it was connected to the early memories of her mom being sick and feeling overwhelmed. That became the first target, and then she addressed her mom's death. After that, memories of her unhealthy rela-tionships were processed along with the recent breakup. The result was the elimination of Ava's fears, and she was able to move on, feeling good about herself. This also directly affected the choices she made in men and what she was willing to put up with, since the sense of safety was now within herself.

IT'S JUST NOT SAFE

Feelings of not being safe show up in hundreds of ways. Perhaps we feel anxious meeting new people or when in new situations. Some people feel that they're inadequate to handle situations, or feel like "imposters" waiting to be found out. Others feel anxious about taking tests because they inappropriately feel "stupid" or incapable—viewing themselves as "failures." Whether the reasons stem from humiliations in school or problems at home, the bottom line is that whenever we're in certain situations, we feel a physical response of fear or anxiety that colors how we view the world and what we're capable of doing. Fears can become worse over time because each experience becomes encoded in our brain and the memory network associated with the problem increases. As we accumulate more actual experiences of blowing a test or withdrawing and being ignored at a party, we can become more and more convinced of our own inadequacy and inability to handle things.

Negative Cognitions

In this section, we'll explore in depth issues related to the second category of negative cognitions, which is called *Lack of Safety/Vulnerability*. These cognitions relate to troubling feelings that involve fear and a lack of safety. While people who have PTSD or phobias may have negative beliefs in any of the three categories, they can most easily identify those in this category since the feelings of anxiety and fear are part of the diagnosis to begin with. In most cases something specific happened that caused a fear reaction, and this experience remains unprocessed—so walking into a similar situation, or even thinking about certain things such as public speaking or snakes, brings up the negative emotions and physical sensations. Most people with PTSD or a phobia are able to identify the actual cause of the fear—such as a rape or a dog bite. For others, the fears have been there so long that they can't remember where they came from. Regardless, with assistance the memory networks encoding the fears can be addressed.

You Can't Outrun It

There is an old American Indian saying that "You can't outrun what's inside you." Wherever we are, wherever we go, the fear remains in our memory networks waiting to be triggered. Sometimes the negative emotions are low grade, and sometimes they are full-blown phobias that cause people to arrange their lives so they don't have to get anywhere near the things that make them afraid. Phobias generally involve a fear of the fear. In fact, some people report they've avoided the activity so long that they no longer know if they actually still fear it. Rather, they are afraid of being overwhelmed by the fear itself if it arises. This is a very appropriate attitude if you've never been able to deal with fear adequately.

In order to address this problem, some forms of therapy focus on teaching the client a number of self-control procedures, some of which you've already learned. They may also use "exposure therapy" or "behavioral experiments" to have the person confront their feared objects or situations, or test their negative beliefs about the dangerousness of the situation, until the anxiety subsides. These are the most extensively researched forms of therapy for phobias. Although the amount of success and relapse rates vary depending on the type of phobia addressed, these therapies are often excellent options. The EMDR research in this area is much less extensive. However, a survey of EMDR clinicians worldwide has reported a high success rate in addressing these problems. In addition, experiences over the past 20 years have also given us more information about the memory network associations in the brain. Basically, in EMDR therapy, the focus of the treatment is processing the memories that cause the fear itself. In other words, going straight to the source.

For most people the original cause of a fear is fairly straightforward. It's directly related to an experience where they were frightened or harmed in some way. If a dog has bitten me, I may become afraid of dogs. For others, a fear in one area can be caused by something else that happened around the same time. For instance, Cheri was afraid of driving and had been for about ten years. It turned out that her phobia started when she was in college and an exchange student in Europe. Shortly after arriving, some new acquaintances invited her to a party. She happily went, hoping for some budding friendships. When she got to the party she saw a bowl of punch. She drank some, began to feel ill, and returned to her apartment. She lay down in bed and started hallucinating all night, out of control. Someone had spiked the punch with LSD.

Imagine the feeling of being alone in a country where you really don't know anybody, and suddenly hallucinating out of control with no family or friends to call on for help. She was terrified, but she weathered the experience. Then, a couple of days later, she was driving to school. A car swerved toward her. Although there was no crash, it triggered that same feeling of being out of control she'd had in her apartment, and the fear transferred to the driving experience. That was the cause of the driving phobia. In addition, the frightening result of the party also gave her the feeling that it wasn't safe to let down her guard around people—since she blamed herself for being too "trusting" in drinking the punch.

Another example was Stacey, who was also in college and began to suspect that her best friend and her boyfriend were having an affair. So she asked them and they said, "No, of course not." She then began to think, "Oh my god, how can I suspect these wonderful people?" But all the while her gut was feeling, "Something's wrong." Ever had one of those? That went on for a while until one day she was on a bus and, while looking out the window, she saw them on the corner in a passionate embrace. Realizing that they'd been lying to her, that they really were having an affair, she became nauseated. She made it to the next stop, ran off the bus, and vomited in the street. That was the experience that led to a full-blown phobia of public transportation. It also gave her the feeling that she couldn't trust anyone.

So for people with negative cognitions in the Lack of Safety/Vulnerability category, there is the feeling that "I'll be hurt if I do. . . . " The hurt can be physical or emotional. It could be that I may crash in a car or a plane, be bitten by a snake or a dog, drown, or any of a thousand other fears—or I may be shamed or deprived or someone will take advantage of me if I do something. For instance, Catherine sought treatment for her long-standing depression and very high anxiety, which was so intense that she could no longer work. She connected her anxiety and depression with her father's violence in the home, especially toward her two brothers. This made sense, but taking a good clinical history can often reveal other hidden memory connections.

During the EMDR history-taking phase, Catherine also mentioned that she couldn't cry, but she didn't know why and couldn't say when it had begun. While processing a memory of her father's bullying, a new memory emerged. She said, "When I was three, I doubled over in church in pain, and I must've passed out, because the next thing I woke up in the pediatric unit at the hospital. It was nighttime, and my mother had left, and I was crying that I wanted my mommy. The nurse said, 'If you don't stop crying, I'm not going to let your mommy come to see you!' That was years ago, but that's the root of me putting the brakes on—I'm afraid of crying. I hid crying, even as a kid. I'd hide under my bed to cry; isn't that weird?"

Fears can be caused by actual events that hurt us physically or emotionally, by hearing about others being hurt, or for some people, watching scary movies as children can also do it. The bottom line is that our fears and lack of safety are embedded in these unprocessed memories— and sometimes what could have been handled easily at the time becomes a long-lasting problem. For instance, Billy presented with an extreme fear of snakes. When he was around seven years old, he discovered a garter snake crawling on his leg. He became frantic. When he ran home scared and hysterical, his mother punished him for "being a sissy." When he lay awake that night, he could feel the snakes crawling up the poles of the bed. For Billy, the negative cognitions from this incident were not just "I'm not safe"—but "I cannot trust anyone." After all, the person he expected to help him had made him feel even worse. The experience also included the feeling that he wasn't good enough to deserve support. All these problems disappeared after processing the memory.

The same was true for Greg, who was in his late 30s and had such a fear of small animals that he couldn't even join his friends for outings or picnics in the park. It turned out that he had been bitten by a small dog when he was about five or six—but the worst part was his father laughing and dismissing the experience, despite cleaning the bloody wound and bandaging it. Minimizing Greg's emotional reactions instead of comforting him locked in not only the fear, but also the feelings of shame and self-blame.

Greg's father made a fairly common mistake. Adults often try to tell jokes or "kid" their friends out of feeling bad. But when children are frightened and come for nurturing, they crave a parent who is attuned to their need. It's important for parents to acknowledge and calm their children's fears lovingly, in a way that makes them feel they are now safe, and they did the right thing by coming to them. This can turn a frightening experience into a building block of resilience and success. Otherwise, it can turn the experience into a lasting source of pain.

Sometimes the treatment of phobias can become complicated because the fear is serving another purpose. That's known as "secondary gain"—where the person is deriving some benefit from the fear. For instance, if I have a client who is afraid of snakes because he was repeatedly told that they were dangerous, or had been bitten, or had a friend who was bitten, then processing the associated memories will generally handle it. However, I once had a client who was the wife of a camping fanatic. She was afraid of snakes, and that kept her from having to go along with her husband. She hated camping for a variety of reasons, but as in other situations in her marriage, she felt she just couldn't say "No." Until we dealt with the memories underlying her inability to stand up for herself, the fear didn't change. Therefore, it's important to ask yourself: Is this condition serving me in any way? If it is, that's an important area to explore.

TRAUMA WITHIN TRAUMA

People who have experienced a major assault—whether through sexual abuse, accidents, natural disasters or war—can end up with PTSD. They can relive the experience over and over in their minds through nightmares, intrusive thoughts or flashbacks—where they actually feel like the event is happening all over again. There is a wide range of symptoms that can occur and the ongoing feelings of fear and lack of control can disrupt relationships with family and friends because of angry outbursts, depression and withdrawal.

One of the purposes of this book is to provide a greater understanding of what makes us tick—and what we can do about it. Another purpose is to help develop more understanding and compassion for those around us. For these reasons, a man who wants to help his fellow combat veterans and a woman who wants to help other sexual abuse survivors are sharing their stories in this section. As I've said before, we are all more similar than we are different. The ways our memories affect us may vary, but none of us is immune from negative feelings, thoughts and physical responses. Millions of people are affected by trauma because of accidents, natural disasters, terrorist attacks and physical or sexual assault. It can happen suddenly for any of us at any time. If these problems don't directly touch on issues affecting you or a loved one, you might want to consider our shared humanity and vulnerability. As we explore these two stories, you might ask yourself: What would it have been like for me in the same situation?

War and Finding Peace

First responders and veterans are similar in being willing to face danger in order to protect and save others. While they give their all, they are often wracked with feelings of guilt and powerlessness. This is often because they demand themselves to be 100% successful 100% of the time, even when they cannot control 100% of the situation. You may have problems that stem from this kind of internal pressure as well. If you are a first responder, a veteran or the family member or friend of one, this section may have special meaning for you. If you are not in any of those categories, then this case may help you have a better understanding of—and compassion for—what our first responders and combat veterans are going through. In addition, if you have any of the symptoms listed here, it can help you learn something more about yourself. Trauma can cause many physical disturbances and once it takes root, it usually doesn't clear up on its own. For people who have PTSD because they have chosen to serve their country in combat or as frontline responders, life can be especially hard, because they often develop feelings of failure. Most often, their symptoms aren't being caused by fear for themselves, but because of the people they might have hurt—or who they couldn't save. While the experiences that occur in war could be enough to have a negative impact on anyone, there can be additional reasons for breaching the emotional defenses of even the strongest warrior. The following example can give you an idea of how much suffering our combat veterans are experiencing—and how intricately woven our memory networks can be.

Hal Walters is a 37-year-old married, combat-decorated Marine Corps Staff Sergeant (SSGT E-6) with more than 11 years of active-duty service. His military primary care physician referred him for treatment due to postdeployment PTSD and major depression disorder symptoms. SSGT Walters related that within a week of returning home from his second and most recent combat tour in Iraq two years ago, he began to experience progressively worsening problems, along with daily intrusive recollections of combat-related events triggered by a wide range of common stimuli—such as the sight of older women, children, and crowded places.

His symptoms included insomnia, anxiety-related nightmares, intermittent crying jags, irritable and depressive moods, stomach problems, chronic fatigue, problems with concentration and memory, feeling socially disconnected, frequent headaches, periods of emotional numbing alternating with intense anger outbursts or seemingly unprovoked crying spells, hypervigilance (feeling tense and on guard), exaggerated startle (jumping at sudden noises), loss of appetite, feelings of exhaustion and profound guilt in relation to multiple war-related memories. All of these are symptoms—alone or in combination—that affect thousands of our warriors. Millions have been affected dating back to earliest recorded time.

Hal had a number of memories that needed to be processed, but one had extra special significance. He was on guard duty and his platoon was forced to open fire when a car barreled down on them. The disabled, smoke-filled, bullet-riddled car rolled to a stop. A few occupants slowly attempted to open the passenger doors. Exiting the rear door was an elderly Iraqi woman, who was mortally wounded and bleeding profusely. She cried out in obvious anguish and pain, as he and his men watched her collapse in spasms. As he told his therapist, other vehicle occupants were all badly shot-up and lay either dead or quietly dying. However, regulations did not permit the soldiers to approach until the explosive and ordnance disposal people had had a chance to inspect the car and ensure it was not a suicide bomb. The elderly Iraqi woman writhed on the ground and moaned loudly for what he reported seemed like hours, but lasted possibly only minutes until she eventually bled to death.

Hal's facial and emotional expression changed dramatically while retelling the horrific incident. He lowered and shook his head in his trembling hands, as he tearfully recollected the ordeal that he reported reliving several times a day (and at night). Although he denied active suicidal thoughts, intense shame and guilt led him to question why he should continue to live. He frequently made references to the elderly nature of the female victim, so his therapist asked him whether she reminded him of anyone else he knew before. He appeared to carefully consider the question and initially answered "No." Then he quickly changed his mind, stating, "Come to think of it, she reminded me of my grandmother." When asked how so, he replied, "My grandmother was from Nigeria, but lived with us for a few years when I was around eight." He paused and then continued. "But she and my mom constantly argued, I mean really argued. Then I remember one day my grandma told me she couldn't live here anymore and was going to return to Africa."

Hal's therapist asked him whether she did indeed return to her home. He replied, "Yeah, she left almost the next day. I remember her crying when she said good-bye to me the day she flew back, and I never saw her again."

"You never saw her again?" his therapist asked.

"Nope, she didn't have a phone and couldn't write and didn't have e-mail. The last I heard about my grandma was about two years after she went home. My mom told me she had been diagnosed with cancer and died." Hal lowered and shook his head. "I should have stopped her from leaving. If I had, she might still be alive." When asked what he meant, he replied, "If her cancer was diagnosed here in the States, she could have gotten treatment here instead of Nigeria, which could have saved her life."

He went on to express his guilt for not intervening between his mother and grandmother and preventing the rupture in the family ties. When asked how he thought his grandmother and the elderly Iraqi woman might be connected, he gazed ahead and said, "I never realized that before, but she was about the same age as my grandma, and in both cases I felt responsible for their deaths."

Hal was asked to concentrate on the stomach sensations and to let his mind go back to the earliest time in his life where he felt those sensations along with feeling responsible or guilty about someone getting harmed. Almost immediately he recalled an outing with his younger brother when he was around six years old and his brother was four. They were walking on rocks near a pond when his brother slipped and hit his head. Hal's hands began to tremble as he told about being "scared" and guilty as his brother cried out loudly with his face covered in blood. He ran home to get his father, who yelled at him and later beat him for not watching out for his brother. This memory and the one with his grand-mother were processed to completion. He was able to recognize how young he had been, and that at six years old he had done his best by running for help. At eight years old, there was nothing he could have done to prevent his grandmother from leaving.

At that point the experience in Iraq was targeted and processed. At the end of the session the SUD was checked, and Hal registered a 1 rating. When asked what kept it from being a zero, he replied, "An innocent old woman died and it will never be a zero. Even though I know I had something to do with her death—I also know that we had no choice. All we saw was a car speeding right toward us that didn't respond to our warnings. If we didn't fire, a lot more people could have been killed. It's one of those tragedies that isn't right, but is a fact of war." As I've said before, processing incorporates what's useful and releases the rest. Veterans don't lose their humanity or the "edge" they might need to survive. But they can let go of the pain of what they've been forced to do in situations they couldn't control.

Another thing to remember is that we all have experiences in our childhood that can make us vulnerable to different kinds of problems. All it takes is some accumulation of later experiences to tip us over. These types of experiences are most notably found in wartime. In fact, the kinds of events that occur during war can be sufficient to deliver a body blow that becomes impossible to recover from alone. Combinations of fatigue, exertion, responsibility, relationships with those who have died, horrific images—the list goes on and on. Wrong time, wrong place, luck of the draw. Whatever the reason, the research is clear—after three months, PTSD is considered "chronic." Symptoms can persist for life if they are left untreated. There can also be delayed reactions where years later something triggers the negative feelings or self-judgment. The bottom line is that the symptoms can emerge at any time. Our enlisted men and women may be returning home with visible or invisible wounds— and deserve our help, understanding and respect. Who among us could have withstood these experiences intact?

PTSD makes life unmanageable. It pushes people into trying to do something to survive the chaos within them. Some people turn to drugs or alcohol, which only makes matters worse. The people who come in for help should be honored for their bravery and willingness to confront their demons. Whether or not there are intrusive thoughts, nightmares or flashbacks of a specific event, if any of the symptoms that SSGT Walters had are part of your life, consider your options. You can keep trying to fight it alone or reach out for assistance, just as this veteran chose to do. You don't have to talk about what happened in detail, and relief may be as quick as 12 sessions away. Resources are listed in Appendix B. Please reach out for help.

Keeping Secrets

For many sexual abuse victims of any age, whether raped or molested, there are often feelings of guilt and shame, along with feelings of lack of safety and power. Rape victims might be made to feel they brought it on themselves—by dressing a particular way or walking down a particular street. These feelings are unjustified. No one has the right to exert sexual power over another in any way. The responsibility for what happened completely belongs with the rapist—just as it belongs to any child molester.

The negative feelings that get locked into abuse victims are symptoms, not reality. As we have seen, the three categories of *Responsibility, Lack of Safety and Lack of Control/Power* help verbalize the negative feelings we have. They are also the labels for the different plateaus of processing that occur with EMDR treatment. Consequently, as with other trauma victims, sexual abuse survivors are able first to put the responsibility on the perpetrator, where it belongs, then lose the sense of fear as the memory is integrated into the appropriate networks so that it takes its place in the past, and are then finally able to experience a sense of power and the ability to make new choices in the present.

The following story is being shared by a molestation victim in hopes of helping others like her, and to assist everyone to recognize some of the warning signs and effects of this type of assault. Nancy's father began abusing her at a very young age—as far back as she could remember until she was 12 years old.

I was 36 years old when I sat in my children's grade school auditorium for a parent assembly on the topic, "Keeping Our Children Safe from Sexual Abuse." As the lecturer described the typical abuser (someone known to the child, someone who gains the child's trust through games that escalate from innocent to invasive), I suddenly burst into uncontrollable tears. I couldn't stop crying and couldn't get up and leave. I felt frozen in place. Although I always remembered my father coming in my room at night and rubbing against me, touching me between my legs, making me promise to keep secrets, until that moment I didn't realize that the patterns of abuse were typical and that I was not alone.

Fear of my father and his control of my body were all a part of everyday life for me as a child. My body seemed not my own. I never dared tell anyone. I believed that my father would kill me or tell my mom, which would result in her leaving us. I didn't know that I had the right to tell him to stop and that what my father did was not my fault. Sometimes I felt he was punishing me for something bad I had done. Other times he convinced me that I'd wanted him to do it. I liked other kinds of attention he gave me, so I felt that maybe it was my fault. The whole time it was happening, I felt as if I was part of something wrong and shameful in which I was hopelessly stuck.

I was in therapy off and on throughout my adult life for depression and anxiety. Although those processes helped, they didn't do enough to free me from my symptoms. I awoke screaming at the slightest noise, I was very alert to danger, real and imagined, I felt haunted by my father, who died when I was a teenager. I was afraid that he could somehow come to life and kill me for telling about the sexual abuse I had suffered. My bouts of depression were severe, rendering me unable to work and only able to carry out the minimal actions necessary to keep life going. My feelings about myself caused me to desperately attach to men who didn't treat me nicely or care for my needs. I had no right to my own body, and intelligence wasn't important. Being attractive and appealing so that someone would want me were all that mattered.

Several years ago, in the middle of another severe depression, a friend of mine recommended EMDR. My new therapist and I set up some safety measures when I focused on painful memories so I knew that I could deal with whatever emotions they triggered. We could stop, put things in perspective, take a break, go slowly. As it turned out, I felt safe with the process immediately and we were able to move rapidly through a number of memories—one per session. We processed through the memories one by one. My feelings and the memories seemed to change spontaneously to better ones. At first, my mother came and rescued me. Later, I found ways to rescue myself. The new images just came up automatically. I can think of the incidents now without feeling *as if it just happened. I know it was a frightening time. I know how I felt, but I don't reexperience those feelings now.*

One of the first memories I worked with was a time when I was five years old, with my father in downtown Chicago. He became angry and walked away from me. I felt lost, helpless, frightened. I didn't know how to find him. We didn't live in Chicago and I had no idea how I could find my way home. That is all I remembered of the incident, but whenever I thought of it I felt cast back through the years to my five-year-old self, abandoned and alone. Over the years, whenever someone was late to pick me up or forgot a meeting, I experienced that same sense of being frightened and abandoned and angry. That's over now.

I don't know the theories behind the ways in which the process impacts people. I only know that it feels as if the traumas of my childhood and the fragile sense of self I had were somehow transformed. What felt dangerous and present and outside my control became a memory within me, no longer looming large outside me.

If you or someone you know is struggling with this type of history, please know that help is available. It's important to remember that the shame and self-blame you are feeling are the SYMPTOMS, not the reality. Remember the example I gave at the beginning of the book about the nursery rhyme? If you hear the words "Roses are red," then "Violets are blue" will pop up, even though it isn't true. Well, feeling shame and self-blame is "Violets are blue"—in spades. Just because you feel it doesn't make it so. It may make it difficult for you to tell your story. But, since the EMDR processing occurs internally, it's not necessary to talk in detail about what happened to you. You can do it at your own pace, in your own time. The self-control techniques in this book can help make life more manageable. But as with PTSD from war, once trauma takes root it generally needs professional assistance to overcome. There is much more to life than simply managing the pain. It's not your fault, and as Nancy said, you're not alone.

WHY CAN'T I CHOOSE?

As we've seen, the things that traumatize us can make us feel fearful and anxious, and also take away our power to choose. In many ways we may not suspect, our life is run by earlier events that push us into doing things that seem to make sense, but are really unhealthy for us. For instance, 67-year-old Susan turned to EMDR therapy to help her because she felt overwhelmed. She was unable to say "No" to anyone. She was very motivated to change, and had already begun to identify some stressors and obligations she could eliminate. However, the way she viewed her relationships with her daughter, granddaughter and husband would be the bigger challenge. "They all need me," she said. Whether it was financial support, crisis intervention or rescuing, she was the go-to gal for too many people—and it was causing her to feel lost and depleted. In conversation with her therapist, she recognized the need to make changes in how she responded to them while staying lovingly involved. But it was easier said than done.

When questioned by her therapist, Susan said that she had no major trauma memories that she was bothered by. "Well, there was that thing that happened with my older cousin, but that can't be anything because I never think about it and when I do now, it's no big deal. Those things happen, and life goes on." She was mildly irritated when her therapist recommended processing this event. "Seems like it would be a waste of time." However, she decided to try to see if anything might come of it. The event was a memory of being raped by her teenage male cousin when she was eight years old. She was surprised by the feelings that came with the processing—hurt, anger, rage and abandonment. Her most striking awareness came from the feeling of violation, along with her desire to please. She knew she did not want her cousin to be mad at her, and he threatened to not play with her again if she didn't comply.

Susan began the follow-up session by declaring she still didn't really know why, but she knew now with great certainty that she would never, never let anyone take advantage of her again. She had, for the previous week, seen more clearly than ever how her family and others in her life had abused her kindness, and she wasn't happy about it. With more processing, Susan went on to have healthier relationships with her family members. She was now comfortable with saying "No" without feeling she'd be rejected for standing up for herself. That's a problem that many of us have. If you are in that category, it would be useful to take a look at what's driving it. Are you being pushed by unprocessed memories that make you feel that way?

On the other end of the spectrum was Benjamin, who shied away from helping others, especially in crisis situations. He was plagued with feeling different from other people, not as empathetic or caring, and not reacting "normally" in times of stress. The Floatback technique brought up an incident where he witnessed a car accident involving some of his friends. He and a couple of buddies saw the crash, so they ran to the car to help. Benjamin tried to assist his friend who was inside, but when he opened the door, she fell out and hit her head on the pavement. She never regained consciousness and died a few days later. He blamed himself because he thought he'd caused her death by not preventing her from hitting her head.

Now, during the EMDR processing, he made comments like "Oh, this is so silly" or "I can't believe I'm doing this" and finally said, "OK, I get the point, it wasn't my fault!" Shortly after that, he moved to another town. Several months later he sent an e-mail to his therapist. He had been in an airport and a woman walking in front of him fell down. He said he dropped his luggage and was the first person to rush up and help her. A few days later it dawned on him that he'd reacted very normally to a crisis. He'd been very concerned about her and had acted in a way he thought other people would respond in that situation, rather than how he'd reacted in the past. He realized that he had related taking action/reacting to causing his friend's death. Now his responses came automatically from processed memories, rather than unprocessed ones. Since he was no longer being pushed by the old stuff, he could choose his own path.

PERSONAL EXPLORATION

Anxiety or fear can come from an experience that caused either physical or psychic pain. It makes no difference. Either source can cause us to develop PTSD symptoms, full-blown phobias, low-grade anxiety or a negative sense of self. The list of negative cognitions we explored in the previous chapter emphasized the feeling "There is something wrong with me." The ones we will deal with in this section are the two other categories, which emphasize lack of safety and lack of control/power.

Lack of Safety/Vulnerability

We've already examined a number of examples having to do with fear and anxiety. If you know you have a phobia or PTSD, you can easily identify which of the negative cognitions (listed on the next page) apply to you. For those of you who don't, or if you want to see if you have any other hot spots in this area, start a new page in your notebook with the heading "Lack of Safety." Be prepared to use your Breathing Shift, Belly Breath or

Safe/Calm Place techniques if you need them. Then write down in your notebook the first thing that comes to mind that completes this sentence:

It's not safe to _____.

Now read through the following list slowly and notice your body reactions. Write down the negative cognitions that seem to relate to you. Once you've finished, if you choose, you can use the Floatback technique you learned in Chapter 4 and identify the present events and memories for your *Touchstone List.*

Lack of Safety/Vulnerability

I cannot trust anyone.
I am in danger.
I am not safe . . . (Fill in your own and/or choose from below.)
   It's not safe to make mistakes.
   It's not safe to feel.
   It's not safe to show my emotions.
   It's not safe to be unguarded.
   It's not safe to assert myself.
   It's not safe to be vulnerable.
   It's not safe to depend upon others.
   I'm not safe unless I am in charge.
   I'm not safe unless I get what I want and need.
   It's not safe to be close.
   It's not safe to love.

These kinds of feelings generally originate from unprocessed experiences that are the hidden source for many reactions in the present. For instance, Max was very angry with his coworker who never followed through on what she said she was going to do. When he processed his recent experience with the negative cognitions "I'm not safe/I can't trust," a past memory connection came up. When Max was a little boy seeing the doctor, he was told the shot he was going to get wouldn't hurt. It hurt. What the doctor said didn't happen. After this memory was processed, Max's anger at his coworker disappeared. The coworker was just a person you could predict would not follow through. Max's past was no longer pushing his present reactions. The fact that an experience with a doctor that happened so long ago was the basis of his problem at work decades later is another example of the intricate, weblike extensions of our memory network. So, if you use the Floatback technique to find the underlying memory, try to just let your mind go wherever it needs to go. Just let whatever happens, happen.

Lack of Control/Power

This category has to do with the ability to make positive choices and exert control in the world. Someone who has successfully eliminated a negative cognition from the previous category may now feel that something, or someone, won't hurt them. This current category concentrates on the negative emotions that say, "I'm not powerful or strong enough to deal with what life gives me" or "I can't be in control of myself or life." In essence, it's about personal power—what psychologists call an "internal locus of control." Meaning that the source of the power is *within* rather than outside of me.

As with the other two categories of negative cognitions, the cause of the negative emotions and beliefs are unprocessed memories of events that give a person the sense of being inadequate or "less than" in some way. For instance, Judy is a 50-year-old woman who was ineffectual in relationships and her career. When she was with her husband, she felt overshadowed and self-conscious. Although she had great creativity, she was having trouble getting her writing career going. One problem was that she felt intimidated, inarticulate, stupid and "slow" when talking to the people who had the kinds of connections that she needed to produce her screenplays. To her therapist, she seemed to live in a chronic state of mild to moderate shame. The negative cognition for her was "I can't succeed." During history-taking, the reason became clear. Her father, who was quite a driven guy, used to set up competitions among his children—everything from word games to sports. As the youngest of four, Judy didn't win very often.

On the opposite end of the spectrum was David, who was driven to excel. His negative cognition was "I have to be perfect" and the stress, combined with the long hours he felt forced to work, was taking a toll on him physically. David's problem was tracked back to a Touchstone Memory that occurred when he was about ten years old. His father worked 12-hour days and was generally exhausted when he got home. His own upbringing and fatigue contributed to a very short fuse. One day, David was completing his spelling homework and his father came in to test him. Although David knew the answers, he was nervous and kept making mistakes—and his father became more and more frustrated. Finally, after another wrong answer, David's father lashed out and smashed his fist through the wall. Although his father laughed about it in later years, for David it was a defining moment. As he explained it, "It could have been my head!" Basically, after that experience, failure wasn't an option, no matter what it took to succeed. He couldn't do less than "everything" or he felt anxious and fearful.

Whether the issue is feeling like you're helpless or you always have to be in control, the underlying reasons can generally be found by examining your memory networks. So begin by identifying which of the negative cognitions in this category are hot for you. We're looking for negative feelings and physical sensations that go along with the belief. For instance, the words "I'm powerless" will generate negative feelings when a rape victim with an unprocessed memory thinks of them—but may have a positive emotion for someone who has completed a 12-Step Program. As you've done before, read the list below slowly and notice your body's response. Write your choices down in your notebook under the heading "Lack of Control/Power." Once again, after you've finished, if you choose, you can use the Floatback technique and identify the recent events and memories for your *Touchstone List.*

Lack of Control/Power

I am not in control.
I am powerless (helpless).
I cannot get what I want.
I cannot stand up for myself.
I cannot let it out.
I cannot trust myself.
I am a failure (will fail).
I cannot succeed.
I have to be perfect.
I cannot handle it.

CHOOSING TO CHOOSE

As I said previously, fear and anxiety may be warning signals that we need to evaluate the situation and decide whether there is real danger, and what we need to do about it. But sometimes the feelings may be the residue of old stuff. If you've been keeping your TICES Log, then you've gotten a broader sample of the kinds of situations that cause you distress. If you've identified your negative cognitions and the memories driving them, then you've gotten a good idea of the kinds of things that are running your show. Phobias, PTSD and other intense fears generally need a therapist's assistance to overcome. In other instances, self-control techniques can help make life more manageable and increase your positive feelings.

SAFE/CALM PLACE ARSENAL

If you've been keeping a list of the current situations and negative cognitions, you can also identify the kinds of negative feelings you often have and add to your collection of techniques. Take a look at your list and see how often certain negative feelings and thoughts arise. If you identified a Safe or Calm Place, you can also pick other feelings and emotions that you can use when you feel upset. If you often feel "I'm not good enough," do you have any positive memories where you felt a sense of accomplishment? If so, use the Safe/Calm Place exercise you learned in Chapter 3 and connect the different positive feelings to other key words and images that you can bring up at will. If you often feel "I'm not lovable," see if you can remember a time when you felt secure—meaning safe and accepted as you are. Use the exercise to make those feelings available to you if you feel triggered.

If you have trouble thinking of any positive memories, this gives you important information. Sometimes they may be difficult to remember, especially if you are feeling depressed. The research shows that when we feel depressed, it's hard to think of anything positive because our brains are primed to bring up only memories that have those downbeat emotions. If that is the case, or if you find that the Safe/Calm Place connections and other techniques are not enough to overcome your negative feelings in different situations, then consider working with a therapist to process the memories that are causing your pain. Guidelines for choosing a therapist are in Appendix B.

We're not responsible for the negative experiences we had as children. However, as adults we are responsible for deciding what to do about them. If you've discovered things about yourself that you would like to change, the question to consider is whether you can accomplish it on your own or whether you need assistance.

I sometimes wonder what the world would be like if we were all brought up in households that knew how to love and cherish and raise us well. Two of my colleagues have a beautiful son named Adam. When he was about three years old, he slipped and fell into the deep end of a swimming pool and started to sink. His father immediately dove in after him and handed him out to his mother at the edge of the pool. It was pretty frightening for everyone involved. But she used some of the techniques you've already learned and dealt with her fear so she could concentrate on Adam. She didn't show how frightened she'd been. She didn't try to laugh him out of his fear. She hugged Adam and kept saying to him, "It's over. You're safe now," while leading him to take slow, deep breaths. They talked about the incident again and again that day; each time she reassured him and led him into the slow, deep breaths.

Then about six months later, when Adam's mother was lifting him out of the bathtub, he looked her straight in the eye, threw his arms tightly around her neck, and said, "I'm safe now" and "I love you, Mommy." He then asked her if she remembered pulling him out of the swimming pool and comforting him. Of course, she said that she definitely remembered the experience and was so happy that he knew that he was safe and protected and loved.

When Adam was six years old, his parents and I were visiting together and stopped at a playground. Adam went up into some tunnels and netting high above. After a while, we realized it was getting late and asked him to come down. He started to come, but moved very slowly and kept stopping. Not knowing what was going on, we called to him again, but he kept moving slowly and stopping. Suddenly we realized what was happening. A little girl, around four years old, whose mother was nowhere around, had managed to climb up to the netting and was afraid to come down. Adam kept urging her to follow him as he moved slowly along, stopping to allow her to catch up. He wouldn't leave her. Finally, when they had made their way down to the ground, he looked her in the eye, patted her on the arm, and said, "It's over, you're safe now." Then he was able to walk away as her mother came running up.

I wonder what the world would be like if we had a whole generation of Adams raised by loving and responsive parents. Little boys and girls who are aware, confident and kind enough to help others instead of making fun of weakness or ignoring those in need. Many of us didn't have childhoods like Adam. But the good news is that it's not too late for any of us to "re-parent" ourselves with the proper assistance.

The Butterfly Hug

While EMDR therapy needs to be conducted with the help of a trained and licensed therapist, you can use one of its components for self-care. You cannot do memory processing, which needs all of the EMDR therapy procedures. But you can try a form of the bilateral stimulation component—tapping—that might be useful to reduce minor anxiety. Researchers theorize that the alternate tapping sets off a relaxation response. However, sometimes it can move your mind into associated negative material. So it's important to monitor the effects.

As I've mentioned in Chapter 3, the Butterfly Hug was developed in Mexico in order to help groups of people do EMDR therapy. You may have used this form of bilateral stimulation before to strengthen your Safe/Calm Place, when you added in the alternate tapping to see if the positive feelings got stronger. As long as you were able to use it successfully, you can also try it when you're feeling stressed or anxious. However, as with the Safe/Calm Place, it's important to monitor yourself to make sure that you don't start bringing up negative memories. As you now know, your memory networks are intricate webs of associations. You need to monitor your reactions so that you don't end up bringing up a memory that is highly disturbing. If you do, it's important to use one of the self-control techniques to close it down. You can choose from the Safe/Calm Place arsenal, Spiral, Paint Can, Cartoon Character, or breathing techniques.

You can experiment by first positioning yourself to do the Butterfly Hug by crossing your arms across your chest with your left hand on your right shoulder and your right hand on your left shoulder. Now bring up something that is causing anxiety at about a 3 SUD. Have you examined why it's there? Is it indicating a problem that needs action? If so, have you decided what to do about it? Then, at this point, it's appropriate to deal with the anxiety directly. So hold an image of the situation in mind and just notice your feelings as you alternately tap each shoulder slowly four to six times. That's one set. Then take a deep breath. If you feel better, then continue for another five sets. If at any time you find it getting worse, or something more negative comes up, then let it go and use your other self-control techniques.

If you found that the Butterfly Hug worked for you now, you can also try alternately tapping your thighs at the same slow speed and for the same length of time. If that also works, then you have another option you can use in different situations. Both these techniques can help you to deal with stress and low-grade anxiety (up to 4 SUD). Just be careful to monitor whether they lessen the disturbance or move it into something more disturbing. Our memory networks are sometimes unpredictable. What works well in one area might not in another. But with the different self-control techniques you are learning, life can become more manageable. The ongoing question for you is whether it is manageable enough— or whether you've set your sights too low in terms of how satisfying and joyful life can be.

THE BRAIN, BODY AND MIND CONNECTION

Body issues take many forms. There's a poem that begins with the lines, "Oh body, my body, my friend and companion. The biggest betrayer my life's ever known." That can sum up the feelings that many of us have. Can't do without it, but can't control it. I want to do something, but my body is doing something else. I've decided to try diving off a high board and my knees are shaking. I go to a party to meet people, but start stammering when I try to strike up a conversation. I want to live my life happily, but I have pain that no doctor can explain. So in this chapter, we'll deal with a wide range of complaints that involve major body issues. These are very common and often very treatable if we examine when the problems started and what was going on at the time. We'll begin by exploring a wide range of conditions that people may believe are purely physical, but might actually be caused by unprocessed memories. We'll end the chapter with both personal exploration and a self-control technique that many people find helpful for pain control.

When psychologists talk about "psychosomatic" issues, they are generally referring to the effect of the "psyche" (the mind) on the "soma" (the body). However, for many people this can feel as if their suffering is being discounted as "It's all in your mind." Actually, it's not. The body's control center is the brain. There is always an interaction of brain, mind and body. Sometimes our body reactions affect our peace of mind. Everyone has had the experience of feeling down when they are sick or overly tired. It's equally true that our state of mind affects our body. There is plenty of research showing that mental stress affects our cardiac, respiratory and immune systems. However, as we explore different possible body/mind issues, let's remember that it's the way memories are stored in the brain that may be directly affecting how we feel and respond both mentally and physically. Even when there is an obvious physical problem, such as a disease or amputation, how we feel about that condition can be influenced by our unprocessed memories. Other times, the symptoms caused by unprocessed memories can masquerade as medical problems.

STOP, YOU'RE KILLING ME

Let's begin with Carl, who suffered from a condition affecting thousands of people. Here's how he explains feeling for the past 30 years:

The symptoms began when I was about 13 or 14 years old. I can't remember exactly when I began feeling sick or what I was doing, but it's been part of my life for a very, very long time. When it hits I get light-headed, shaky, sweaty and dizzy to the point where I can't walk or function. Eventually I throw up. Throughout my life I've been to many medical doctors who all had theories, but nobody had the answers. The only thing I could do to feel better was go to sleep for a couple of hours or so. As I discovered, there are many medical conditions that show these symptoms. Nothing the doctors gave me helped.

As I grew older, began my college career, and eventually got married, these symptoms continued to affect and control my life. I would get sick playing sports, taking tests, public speaking, dating, interviewing, going to parties, etc. This "monster" was controlling my life and I had no answers. This sickness has put a great deal of strain on my marriage and my relationship with my children, to the point where divorce seemed to be a viable option. As the children have grown and have been involved in various activities (sports, music, etc.), it began to affect my relationship with them also. I coached my son's baseball team for a couple of years but I had to stop because I couldn't take the stress and I would get sick almost every game. Even after I stopped coaching I couldn't even go to his games to watch without getting sick. One day I overheard my son talking to my wife and he said that he "wanted a new dad" because I got sick too much. This hurt and made me realize that I needed to figure something out NOW.

After 30 years of suffering, Carl discovered that he had a panic disorder—and was able to eliminate the symptoms by processing the memories driving the physical reactions. Some of the memories involved moving to a new school and pressures to play sports to fit in. People can be traumatized when they first experience a panic attack because they feel very sick or feel that they are dying. Just as we examined in the previous chapter, the feelings of fear can be locked into many childhood memories, which get triggered by a variety of stressful situations in the present. What complicates the picture even further is that the brain responds to the fear by pumping the body up, getting ready to deal with some kind of threat. But the dominant feelings include fear and powerlessness. So now the body reactions also feel out of control. The physical sensations, which include heart palpitations, dizziness, shortness of breath—all for no apparent reason—then become a source of terror and the thought "I'm going to die from this" can also get locked into the memory network. Where do you run when it feels as though your own body is killing you? Then worrying about when another set of out-of-control physical sensations will hit adds to the stress, which adds to the body reactions, and it becomes a vicious circle. On top of that, the physical sensations are real. Saying it's "all in your mind" makes no sense when you are throwing up and passing out. So people often get caught up in years of traveling from one medical doctor to another looking for solutions, just as Carl did. But the brain/body/mind connection holds the answers, and freedom can come from targeting the unprocessed memories driving the reactions.

Many kinds of childhood events that feel uncontrollable can cause long-lasting fear responses. For instance, the research on panic disorder reports that more than half the people suffering from it were separated from their parents sometime in childhood or adolescence—through death, divorce or some other reason. Children can be badly affected, because the feeling of being abandoned is common in these kinds of experiences. The child wonders "What did I do wrong?" and can always find something to explain it. There is also the natural feeling of being alone and afraid when one of the people who was supposed to love and protect you is gone. All of these feelings can get locked into the memory networks, and when there is enough stress later in life, these unprocessed memories can get triggered as out-of-control body reactions.

Breathless

We've seen in previous chapters how nonnurturing parenting styles can be the source of many problems. There are not only emotional consequences for children, but there may be negative physical consequences as well that can begin very early. For instance, childhood asthma can sometimes be traced back to a lack of maternal bonding. Little Gianna was only seven months old and was already diagnosed with asthma. She had shortness of breath daily, often needing a rescue inhaler, and woke her mother at least four nights a week because she couldn't breathe. She was on two medications, but still needed ER visits. The physicians rated her overall health as a "D" on a scale of A to F.

Her mother, Juanita, believed that Gianna was asthmatic because it ran in her family. Three nephews, one niece and two aunts were severely asthmatic. On her husband's side, seven cousins were asthmatic. However, we have found that childhood asthma is often associated with maternal stress. What Juanita told her therapist fit the pattern. She came from a strict, religious family and had gotten pregnant before she was married. She was "bummed out" and hid it from her family. She said that her "heart ached." When she told her family, they were so upset that they did not come to the wedding. She felt horrible about causing her parents so much disappointment.

Juanita was scared and depressed all the time. She was heartbroken that her family didn't support her. She had a difficult labor, and the baby was delivered by C-section. Gianna was immediately removed from her mother, and when she was returned three hours later, was not able to nurse. Juanita said that when she first held the baby, she did not feel love, just "scared." She felt unable to really connect with Gianna either emotionally or physically. Because of insurance issues, she was rushed out of the hospital before she was ready to be discharged, and her husband had to return to work sooner than she wanted.

During three processing sessions, Juanita's memories were targeted, including the shock of finding she was pregnant, her family's reaction, the sadness and fear through the pregnancy, and the labor and delivery—including her sadness when her daughter was not with her and the fear when she first held her. Then during processing she visualized a new birthing experience, this time without fear. She felt excited when she imagined finding out she was pregnant—and she experienced what it felt like to be thrilled throughout her pregnancy. She wept with joy. Next, she imagined Gianna being born without a C-section. They stayed together after the birth, and she cried when she experienced how this felt. She then stayed in the hospital as long as she wanted. Everything went beautifully.

At the end of the session, Juanita was asked to go home and rest for the remainder of the day. When she returned the following week, she announced that to her great surprise, she felt uncommonly happy. What's more, her newfound sense of well-being and love seemed to have affected her daughter. Gianna's asthma had disappeared—no daytime or night-time symptoms, no wheezing with play. She was not showing any need for the medication. Everything seemed perfect. One year later, Gianna was still symptom-free.

Mind, Brain and Body

The bottom line is that a wide range of emotional and physical sensations can be the result of unprocessed memories. As we saw in Chapter 5, they can cause a lack of bonding that prevents the maternal feelings of love and nurturing—which goes along with a physical sense of being numb or empty. At the other end of the spectrum, they can cause intense physical reactions. The physical sensations generated by panic disorder, and those that accompany childhood asthma, are real sensations the body is producing in response to a feeling of danger. The feelings of danger that are encoded in the unprocessed memories stored in the brain can be triggered by events in the present.

Although these intense feelings and uncomfortable physical sensations are caused by unprocessed memories, it's not "all in your mind"—since your brain sends out signals to the rest of your body. The brain is part of the body and is the source of all our body responses. Conditions such as panic disorder and childhood asthma can be physical responses to the physical reality of improper memory storage. It's an important point to consider if numerous attempts at a medical intervention don't achieve results. Perhaps it's not purely a medical condition, and a different kind of intervention is required. It wouldn't take very long to investigate if unprocessed memories are at the core of the problem.

THE BURDENS OF THE PAST

One of the participants in the controlled study I published in 1989 reported to me that the treatment eliminated a gagging sensation that she'd experienced several times a week since she'd been orally raped. Not long after that, I was working with another client named Beth to deal with her driving phobia. She'd had a couple of car accidents and we used them as targets for processing. During one of the sessions, Beth said she felt a pulling sensation near her back, which suddenly released. Afterward, she told me that the feeling was the same as the one that had sent her to a chiropractor almost monthly. She'd never connected it to the driving accident that happened years before in which she'd been physically injured. After that session, she never experienced the sensation or the need to visit the chiropractor again. Another client's hunched-over posture spontaneously straightened up as we processed memories of childhood humiliations. These kinds of experiences make it clear that the sensations weren't in their "minds"; they were in their brains and were being felt in their bodies.

Banishing Phantoms

With aches and pains that come and go, it's sometimes difficult to pin down where they originated and why. But nowhere has it been more puzzling than in cases of phantom limb pain. It has been estimated that in the United States alone, there are approximately 1.6 million people who have lost limbs due to accidents, war or disease—about the same percentage of the population as in other developed countries. Land mines cause thousands of limb losses worldwide, mostly for civilians, with the majority being children. About 80% continue to feel their missing limb, and more than half of those are reported to have chronic, often intense, pain.

It's very sad to think of the numbers of people who are needlessly suffering and who think they must be crazy since they feel pain—but there's no limb there. Many of these victims have been told "It's all in your mind"—since the body part is gone and painkillers have no effect. At one time some physicians felt it might be nerve damage and so surgeons tried either severing parts of the spinal cord or cutting up the remaining portion of the limb trying to find a "healthy" nerve. That didn't work either. Now there is a greater understanding of phantom limb pain and scientists view the problem as centered in the way the brain changes in order to organize the amputation experience. Through the use of EMDR therapy, we have also discovered that the phantom limb pain is simply one of the sensations that can be stored in the unprocessed memory of the injury.

Phantom limb pain is different for every person, because it contains the sensations that were experienced at the time of the event. If someone's foot was crushed, or an arm was ripped off, those are the sensations the person can experience, along with all of the pain from the medical procedures that followed. For example, Jim was an active duty Marine whose leg was amputated because of injuries from a motor vehicle accident. He had classic phantom limb pain. This trained, stoic Marine was asked to describe his various pains and the intensity levels on a 10-point scale. Along with feelings of "itching" (3) and persistent "tingling like when your leg falls asleep" (5), he had:

- Dull aching pain—6

- Daily shooting pain—8

- Radiating pain from (phantom) foot to thigh—8

- Severe cramping—9

- Weekly excruciating "sawing" pain—10

Imagine the effects of dealing with this—and no relief in sight. He came into treatment with no real hope of relief from the pain, but in an attempt to deal with the other symptoms related to the accident, including full-blown PTSD with daily intrusive thoughts, hypervigilance (always on the alert for danger), difficulty driving, depression, anxiety, irritability, difficulty sleeping, little energy, guilt, persistent depressed-anxious-irritable mood and insomnia. He felt hopeless about the future and had a hard time being around people because he thought they viewed him as a "freak."

Since Jim was being discharged and sent back to his hometown, he was only able to receive four sessions of EMDR therapy. Nevertheless, during these sessions he made great progress. During the reprocessing sessions, his targets included the memory of sitting on the ground with his leg nearly detached trying to stem the loss of blood. Despite the short amount of treatment time, his PTSD and depression resolved. In addition, all the pain sensations disappeared, except for a tingling sensation at a 2–3 level, which he said was easy to ignore. During processing, Jim summarized his new feeling of personal resilience with the motto "Steel bends and expands, but doesn't break." He also reported a spontaneous image of himself emerging—seeing himself walking confidently with a new prosthesis along with feeling "strong and powerful."

As with Jim, some cases of phantom pain are very clear-cut. We process the memory of the accident, the current triggers and the person's fears about the future. However, it's not always that easy. For instance, a case in Germany was quite complex. A drunk driver hit Alger's motorcycle. His leg was practically pulled off his body and he suffered a number of internal injuries. He was in so much pain that the physicians put him in a medically induced coma after amputating his leg. Although he tried various rehab programs, nothing worked and he continued to suffer intense phantom pain—10 out of 10—for the next 8 years. When he entered rehab again for another try, he encountered a psychiatrist who treated him using EMDR.

It took nine processing sessions to eliminate Alger's pain. In addition to the memory of the motorcycle accident, he needed to process the guilt and loss he felt because of his wife's miscarriage when she heard of his accident. There was also the memory of a visit by a priest at his hospital bed who told him that "God always watches everything and will protect everyone." He remembered feeling anger and a lasting sense of guilt that went along with the thought "I'm not good enough to be protected by God." At the end of that session Alger recognized that he had done nothing to deserve punishment, and he needed to direct his energy toward building a new life. After a couple of other processing sessions based on the scene of the accident, the pain completely disappeared and remained gone—as confirmed by his therapist 18 months, and then 5 years, later.

The bottom line is that although Jim and Alger's physical pain had remained stored in their brains for as long as eight years, it was eliminated after memory processing. These are not isolated cases, as researchers from four different countries have published articles about successfully treating phantom limb pain using EMDR. While there certainly are times when there is serious nerve damage or another type of organic injury, in a great many cases the pain is simply part of the stored memory. For that reason, phantom pain can be felt in different parts of the body. As another example, many women who have had a mastectomy can be troubled by phantom breast pain. As long as the memory of a surgery remains "stuck," there can be phantom pain sensations at the surgical or injury site that may not disappear on their own over time. For the same reason, other people may continue to have feelings of pain long after their wounds have healed from being burned or assaulted. In these cases the pain sensations of the trauma may still be present in the memory networks. If these feelings exist for you, it may be worthwhile to explore whether processing the memory relieves your suffering.

From Head to Foot

Other types of unexplained body pains, including headaches, can also be the result of unprocessed memories. For instance, one of the sexual abuse victims I treated reported that the daily headaches she'd experienced for years cleared up after her EMDR reprocessing sessions. These kinds of reports are quite common. For example, a highly active and successful tour guide used to get migraines every couple of weeks that would lay her up for two days. She had gone to a neurologist, had had brain scans, and had taken every migraine medication in the book, but nothing seemed to help. Her therapist noted that she gave 150% to all her work and was a bit of a perfectionist. Sure enough, it became clear that the day or night before a migraine hit, she had the feeling that she'd done something wrong. Together, they targeted the memories that were feeding the feelings of "I'm a disappointment" and "I'm not good enough," and the migraines disappeared. Another client had gotten headaches every Sunday night since he was eight years old. It turns out that his parents separated around that time and he had to spend every weekend with his dad, returning home every Sunday night to his mom's. From processing the experience of his parents' separation, it was clear that the headaches were an expression of the tension he felt going between his parents' households. So if you or a loved one is suffering with headaches, through processing it may not take long to find out if they are caused by stress or are the remnants of an old memory.

Please remember that even if there was originally a physical cause, it might be useful to check on the source of continued pain. One last example should suffice, just to be clear that the effects of the stored pain can take many forms. A 45-year-old social worker had been driving a car involved in a head-on collision a year before she came in for therapy. Trisha experienced flashbacks, feelings of helplessness, nightmares and intrusive thoughts as well as crippling back and leg pain that affected her ability to function. She needed a walker and dragged her right leg when she walked. The fact that her husband was also injured in the accident intensified her guilt and the feelings that the accident was her fault. During the session that targeted the accident, Trisha saw the image of the headlights coming toward her and her right leg flew straight out as if she were braking. It held that position during the processing, as she realized she had done everything she could. With that, she reported a "healing of the helplessness," a "healing of the pain." At the end of the session, she stood up and walked out of the office unassisted.

This is another example of phantom pain. Trisha's inability to walk had been real. The pain had not allowed her to do it. Although the original cause of the pain was gone, the sensations remained stored in the unprocessed memory of the accident. As with pain that doesn't go away after certain types of surgery, it's another example of how stored memories sometimes show up as physical symptoms.

I CAN'T FEEL A THING

As we've seen, the sensations of an experience stored in our memory networks can produce feelings of pain. They can also be responsible for us not feeling anything—even those feelings we'd like to have. This is a common situation in sex therapy. People feel love for their partners; they want to feel close and be intimate—but they don't have sexual feelings. For some reason, they're blocked. Again, often the memories of a past experience are causing the problem. For example, Bill was referred for EMDR therapy because he was sexually impotent with his partner. His condition tracked back to his parents' divorce when he was six years old. His difficulty came from his mother telling him at the time that he was doing a bad job of replacing his father. Of course, at six years old that wasn't his job. But as we know, young children take on the blame for their parents' flaws. And now, as an adult, his mother's recent illness, which caused her to move into a nursing home, had triggered his guilt, the memory of her disappointment with him, and her words that he was "not being a man." His "impotence" was a physical expression of his feelings of inadequacy about taking care of his mother. During processing, his feelings went from "I'm inadequate" to "I'm fine as I am," and his sexual feelings and abilities returned.

While Bill's problems were triggered by something happening in the present, sometimes sexual problems can be very severe and long-lived. At 34 years old, Sandi was in a sex therapy group for women who were unable to experience sexual arousal or orgasm. She was very much in love with her boyfriend but wasn't able to be intimate. When a group member asked her when she last felt like being sexual, she answered, "Never!" and became very upset.

The therapist offered her individual sessions with EMDR and using the Floatback technique brought up the memory of her first dating experience when she was about 15. Her date had brought her home and as they stood by her front door, their lips met in an innocent first kiss. She remembered just feeling "tingly" for the first time, when her father violently threw open the door and called her a "slut." She immediately shut down and for the next 20 years had not had any sexual feelings. After processing she regained that connection, including the ability to orgasm. The door that had slammed shut her sexual feelings was finally reopened.

Thousands of people suffer from symptoms that masquerade as medical conditions. These can sometimes be identified easily as the result of a single memory, because the lines from one to the other are clear. As in the case of Sandi, something happened and that started her inability to experience sexual feelings. In other instances, it's more complicated because of the many factors that are involved. Some problem seems to be caused by a medical condition. The person has had it before, but it went away. Now, many years later, it comes back. Medical treatments aren't helping and physicians are sure it's just a relapse. It makes perfect sense, but it may not be true. In most instances, people aren't looking for answers to their physical problems when they come in for EMDR therapy. They simply want relief from other emotional symptoms. However, as we've seen, our memory networks are complex and the effects can be far-reaching.

Aaron was 50 years old when he came to therapy to deal with memories of a long-ago student protest of the Vietnam War. He had tried to keep the peace between the students and the police, but in the chaos he'd been beaten and clubbed all over his body. This put him into the hospital for a long time with painful head injuries and numbness in his legs, but he'd recovered after extensive rehab. Now, more than 30 years later, the numbness had come back. For the past 18 months, he'd had to use a walker because of the lack of feeling in his legs. His physicians had diagnosed neuropathy—numbness caused by damaged nerves from his original injury. However, this isn't what motivated him to seek treatment. He'd finally come in for therapy because since US troops had moved into Iraq, he'd been getting flashbacks of his experiences as a Vietnam War protester.

While processing the memory of his beating, other associations came up. He shared something with his therapist that he'd never told anyone else because he was afraid they would think he was crazy. He said that sometimes he thought that maybe he'd lived a past life where he had died in a concentration camp. He couldn't come up with any other explanation for the memories, because he'd had a lifetime of flashbacks and nightmares with all the vivid and gory details of living and dying in one of the camps. He felt powerless, unable to move around, maneuver or do anything to change the horror around him. When the image of being in the camps was targeted, after a few sets of eye movements, Aaron gasped and said, "Oh my god, it isn't me—it's my uncle's memories!" His experience of his uncle's stories, where he saw himself in the situation and actually felt, smelled, tasted and heard everything so vividly and clearly, had come to feel like his own. This is a perfect example of "vicarious traumatization" where people can develop full-blown PTSD from just hearing about an event. It's very common when children are young. They can see something on television, and because they feel bad inside, it feels like it's happening to them.

Aaron had been only four years old when his Uncle Hershel arrived in the US. He was a survivor of a death camp and upon his liberation by Russian forces, Aaron's parents sponsored him to come and live with them. Crowded together in a small apartment, Hershel shared Aaron's bedroom. In order to help protect his nephew, to prevent history repeating itself, to make sure he never forgot what could happen, his uncle recounted many horrible stories of his time in the camps. Suffering from his experiences, he told stories of the daily struggles, fear and sudden deaths over and over again.

Aaron had taken in these stories as his own. Years later, as he processed the memories, he gained insight into how they connected with his own decision-making through his adulthood. He began to see his neuropathy as a symbol of powerlessness, paralysis in life, and inability to maneuver in his world. These were stories and beliefs he had absorbed from his uncle, and he began to realize they did not need to define him. He realized that the feelings of helplessness he'd had when he was beaten during the Vietnam protest had been retriggered by the invasion of Iraq. When those memories of the beatings were activated, the neuropathy he'd experienced at the time also came back. All of these experiences had also been connected to his uncle's stories of being powerless in the concentration camp.

Over a year's time, Aaron and his therapist targeted the memories from the Vietnam War era, the stories he'd heard about the concentration camps, and his difficult relationship with his parents. As his memories were reprocessed, he began to use a cane, and at his final session he was walking without assistance. He was able to maneuver again within his world, free of the crippling memories. It is clear that we can absorb many things in life that aren't our own.

If you have puzzling medical symptoms, there is a possibility that the physical problems are in the brain's memory networks—not the part of the body that is hurting or numb. The feelings connected with phantom pain or numbness are absolutely real. They may come from sensations stored in our memory networks, but there is no difference between how we experience these past sensations and a current medical condition. For instance, if someone pricks your numb hand with a pin, you won't feel it whether it is true neuropathy caused by damaged nerves or a lack of feeling caused by old unprocessed memories. If you have unexplained physical conditions, it might be a worthwhile avenue to explore.

THE CRACKED MIRROR

In the previous section, we dealt with physical symptoms that come from our memory networks. However, there are a wide variety of "body issues" that can bring a person in to therapy. While many of us might wish we could change something about ourselves, some people are intensely troubled by their appearance. They look at themselves and see parts of their bodies as misshapen or ugly. Sometimes they are diagnosed as schizophrenic or paranoid because their views are interpreted as delusions. No one else sees anything wrong, but the person is convinced of it. The results range from avoiding people, to unnecessary surgeries, to suicide attempts. For instance, Stephanie hadn't been able to work for two years because she thought her coworkers were contemptuous of her. She was sure she smelled because of excessive sweating, even though she bathed twice a day, frequently changed her underwear, and used lots of powder and deodorant. She couldn't bear to be in social situations because she thought people were talking about her.

Over the past 15 years she'd had a number of hospitalizations because of thoughts of suicide and was on three different medications. None of it helped. The last straw for Stephanie was finding a can of deodorant near her workstation. She became so overwhelmed with shame, believing it was a comment about her odor, that she deliberately overdosed on sleeping pills when she went home and needed to be hospitalized yet again. During her EMDR therapy she remembered when her problem began. She was 12 years old and she'd brought in food as her teacher had instructed for her Friday cooking class. Unfortunately the class was cancelled. Returning to school on Monday, she went to her gym locker and took out the bag she thought contained her gym clothes. When she opened it, the room was filled with the odor of rotting fish—the food she'd forgotten and left over the weekend after the cancelled cooking class. Her schoolmates made fun of her, accusing her of dirty underwear. Then she was sent to the principal, who scolded her for poor hygiene. She ran home in tears and couldn't bring herself to return for a week. Then, a couple of years later, she'd gone to a doctor who told her she had the sweat glands of a man.

Stephanie had suffered from her belief for 30 years because these earlier experiences remained unprocessed. After three processing sessions the symptoms disappeared and were still gone at a five-year follow-up. For Stephanie, as for many of us, the cause of the symptoms may not be "major traumas" such as natural disasters or physical assaults. They can often be humiliations that occur at a tender age. Adolescence is a very vulnerable time and being made a laughingstock can leave lifelong scars. Stephanie's treatment took three sessions, but she didn't remember the critical event until the last one. The initial targets were more recent experiences of her believing that people were disgusted by her smell. But these memory networks are all connected. So even if you can't remember an early event that caused your problems, it can be worth the exploration. It may be the doorway to freedom from the symptoms.

These same types of memories can be the basis of feelings that cause people to have eating disorders—looking at themselves and believing they are too fat when everyone else around them recognizes that they are wasting away. There are numerous reports of people not being able to eat because of careless remarks made by loved ones during their adolescence. Or choking feelings caused by earlier memories of childhood eating accidents or abuse. While EMDR therapy is not a cure-all, it can help people to regain control over their bodies through processing the memories of experiences that block a healthy and adaptive lifestyle.

People can have many kinds of negative beliefs about their appearance that don't make any sense to the people around them. For example, men can be extremely self-conscious about their thinning hair, spending hours in front of the mirror trying to get it right or having intrusive thoughts of being bald. These can be signs that there is an unprocessed memory pushing their view of themselves. Sometimes the memories of being insulted are clear. Sometimes they're caused by a friend's innocent remark. In Marla's case, she suffered for 24 years with the belief that she was covered with unsightly hair because of a remark that an aunt made about her underarm hair when she was a teenager. The problem became so bad that she wasn't able to go out without plucking out every visible hair—spending hours in front of the mirror daily. Three sessions of processing eliminated the belief and she was able to go swimming with her daughter, happily wearing a bikini, for the first time in her life. As I've said before, it doesn't take long to find out if unprocessed memories are contributing to the problem.

I KNOW SOMETHING'S WRONG, RIGHT?

Many people believe there is something physically wrong with them and spend endless hours searching for answers and diagnoses. While friends and family often dismiss them as hypochondriacs and try to wave their fears away, it rarely works. Sometimes the reasons can be rooted in real illness and loss. For example, becoming overly concerned with getting sick—thinking every cough is an indication of lung cancer because a person previously had cancer or lost a close relative or friend to the disease. Sometimes the problem is caused by a completely unsuspected experience. Whatever the reason, it's important to address the fear and anxiety—not only because it can make life miserable, but because the continued stress can have a negative physical effect as well.

Make It Go Away

Jamie came into therapy after a bout with cancer. She reported that two years prior to the diagnosis she had a growing but unconfirmed suspicion that she had breast cancer, which her doctors considered "irrational" and treated with anxiety medication. Despite self-exams and yearly mammograms, her cancer wasn't caught until it was extremely advanced. Happily, she was successfully treated. But while her tumor marker test was now normal, she was not experiencing the sense of relief she had expected. Instead, she felt a free-fall sensation of panic and a "knowing" that "I'm going to die." It was triggered most severely when she saw signs on local buses that said "Early Detection Saves Lives" during Breast Cancer Awareness Month. She felt anxious, hopeless and frustrated—stating that even if she never experienced a cancer recurrence, she would always have the fear of its return. She didn't know how to *live* now that she had *survived*. Fear of cancer was steadily becoming worse and worse.

Focusing on the current trigger of the bus ads and using the Floatback technique with her clinician brought up the moment of her diagnosis.

She'd had that same feeling of panic and sense of certain death. This is very common with cancer patients. There is the shock of the diagnosis itself, which is often combined with something the physician said or didn't say. Within her first EMDR processing session, Jamie's SUD dropped from an 8 to a 1.

One week later Jamie no longer experienced feelings of panic or the sense of "I'm going to die" in response to the signs. Reevaluation of the memory revealed a SUD of 1, with no emotion associated with the memory, but an uncomfortably hot sensation in her chest. Targeting that brought the emergence and processing of burning sensations in her amputated breast, imagined scenes of her breast being removed during surgery, and the first time she saw her angry stapled scar in the mirror. The burning sensations increased, and then cleared through her arm, chest, neck and head—with no further phantom breast sensations following that session. The positive cognition that emerged was "I'm a tough cookie. As scary as it was, I knew I had the strength to get where I am now. I made it." It felt completely true. When Jamie reported this, she burst into tears of relief, stating, "I had imagined I wouldn't be able to believe that until ten years out!"

During the next session, Jamie identified a belief that she had brought the cancer on herself. Memories of numerous childhood experiences, frozen in their original form with the negative cognition "It's all my fault," were processed and cleared over the course of two sessions. She completed the therapy with a solid belief that "I didn't do anything wrong—this thing just happened" as well as an energized sense that "I have something big to offer." Seven years after her diagnosis all tests indicate that Jamie continues to be cancer-free. She no longer experiences the anxiety that she used to have when she went for yearly mammograms. In addition to resolving the overwhelming fears of recurrence,

Jamie developed a much greater sense of trust in her body, in her intuition, and in her strength to weather whatever life might bring.

These kinds of results are extremely important in many ways. For one, being trapped in the fear of death does not allow us to enjoy life. Those who have faced a disease such as cancer, heart attack or stroke have the choice to fully reenter life or to continue to live in death's shadow. There is no separation between mind and body. In addition to poisoning our present, constant emotional turmoil can also have a negative effect on our physical health. Research is clear that depression and trauma symptoms are associated with an increased likelihood of recurrence or death among people who have suffered a heart attack. Happily, a recent study has shown that only eight sessions of EMDR were able to effectively treat the psychological distress of those who had just had a heart attack. Another study of children suffering from PTSD for more than three years after a hurricane found that they had fewer visits to physicians in the year following EMDR treatment. So if you are not able to deal with your depression or anxiety with the self-control techniques in this book, consider having the trauma processed. And it is a trauma. When we feel that our bodies can't be trusted, or are out of control, it's time to do something about it.

Whether It's Wrong or Right

As we've seen, when we become fixated and overly concerned with how our bodies are responding, the culprit is generally unprocessed memories that are running our show. But sometimes, the feelings from the unprocessed memories that get locked in are not fear, but relief.

Pam was 42 years old when she came in for therapy after years of physical illnesses and accidents. She was in chronic pain and complained of not feeling fully alive. At ten years old, parts of her body had become paralyzed. Doctors could find nothing wrong and told her parents they thought this was psychosomatic. When they got home after the doctor's appointment, her parents tried to get her to "snap out of it." But she spent a night screaming in pain.

It turned out the doctors were wrong. The next morning, Pam's parents took her to the hospital. New tests led to emergency surgery. When she awoke, her mother told her that a cancerous tumor had been removed from her brain. At ten years old, she was happy to hear she had cancer because her family finally believed her. The experience locked in the feeling of "I have to have a diagnosis to be acceptable." These types of experiences can lead many to feel they cannot get people's attention or nurturing unless they are ill. For others, being sick is the only way they can stop taking care of everyone else, or say "No." Either way, unprocessed memories are generally the basis of these problems.

At other times, the cause of the problem involves people who we've only seen once, will never see again, and who have gone on their merry way never even knowing the harm they've done. What's more, they'd probably be horrified to find out the problems they'd caused. For instance, Rita was a 19-year-old college freshman on school break and about to leave for Brazil to study for a semester. Her mother wanted her to have EMDR therapy before she left because of Rita's fears and anxiety. She was healthy, but would "freak out" and obsessively call her mother for reassurance whenever she had a cold or any minor symptom. So her mother wanted to make sure she was OK before leaving the country. A Floatback technique revealed that at age eight, Rita had been taken to the emergency room to be treated for a dog bite. The staff began joking back and forth about her dying from the wound. Although she now understood that they were kidding her, it was clearly locked into her memory networks and she'd been concerned about dying ever since.

Now there are certainly times when there is something very wrong. EMDR therapy is not going to take away a physical condition. For instance, there are thousands of children diagnosed as suffering from Attention Deficit Hyperactivity Disorder (ADHD) who are now on medication. If it is indeed an accurate diagnosis, this is an innate neurological condition and EMDR will not take it away. However, many of the symptoms of ADHD are exactly the same as the ones a child can have after a disturbing or traumatic experience. For instance, Bradley's mother thought he was suffering from a head injury because he'd fallen in the playground the same week the symptoms began, starting with bed-wetting and sleepwalking. Here's how she describes some of the other changes he went through:

As the weeks wore on, the situation deteriorated. Bradley, normally a happy, social, bright boy, became sullen, anxious and easily angered. He would no longer stay alone in a room, not even to take a bath. As a home-schooled student, he has always been bright and focused, easy to teach. He became extremely distracted and fidgety, unable to sit still for even the simplest task. He cried easily and had negative, intrusive thoughts. He would frequently tell me that he "couldn't get the bad thoughts out" of his head. He started lying. His hands began to shake all the time. I had several friends ask me what was wrong with my son. Even his swim coach noticed a marked decrease in his attention span during practice and at meets. His racing times had inexplicably gotten significantly worse, and he looked strikingly awkward and uncoordinated—like he had somehow forgotten how to swim.

It turned out that watching the movie *Predator* had traumatized six-year-old Bradley. The fall was merely a coincidence. When that memory was processed his symptoms disappeared. Many of these problems are also found in children with ADHD. However, it appears that a large number of children are being misdiagnosed with this condition, when the distractibility, conduct problems, irritability and short attention span are the result of unprocessed memories. So if children in your life have any of these symptoms, it might be a good idea to seek professional assistance to see if there are any disturbing experiences pushing them.

EMDR therapy will not eliminate injury, toxin or genetically caused brain deficits. However, in the case of actual ADHD, EMDR can be used to process the memories of failures and childhood teasing and humiliations that often go along with that condition. This can reduce the symptoms, cutting down on the need for medication. Likewise, EMDR researchers have recently reported on cases of people with intellectual disabilities, including some diagnosed with autism. After processing their memories, not only were the trauma symptoms removed, but the caregivers also reported that the people's social and cognitive functioning improved. They took up activities more readily, showed increased independence and learned new skills. For instance, one 54-year-old man who had been diagnosed with autism at 3 years old has spent his life in institutions since the age of 5, sometimes in isolation because of physical aggression. He said that since therapy, *"I feel more relaxed, less gloomy, friendlier, more lighthearted, not so fanatic anymore."* Another intellectually disabled 22-year-old man lives in a group home for people with physical disabilities and was diagnosed with both autism and cerebral palsy. He summarized the changes he felt by saying, *"I have got back my power."* Even with a condition caused by an inborn neurological problem, symptoms can be improved if unprocessed memories are involved.

It is also important to keep in mind that we are learning new things every day. For instance, research has recently indicated that thousands of children may be misdiagnosed with ADHD simply because they started school at an earlier age and are being compared to the older children in their class. Since they are younger, they may be less attentive or unable to keep up. That means they are being needlessly labeled and medicated. It also means that the many failures and bullying experiences that can go along with the situation may need to be processed. Please remember that the same problems and causes apply if you are an adult. Whatever your age, unprocessed memories may be the actual cause of your symptoms, or may be making the problems worse.

Sometimes there is a physical condition that simply won't change. In those cases we can deal with our feelings about it. Many people with physical injuries feel disfigured and shy away from life. Often, fear and guilt become locked in when they try to understand what happened to them. But as an acid burn victim from Bangladesh exclaimed after processing, "The shame is his, not mine." Another acid burn victim in India, who was blinded in the attack by her husband's first wife, is no longer fearful. Although previously illiterate, she has learned Braille and has taken over raising her children.

Not only is there a way to rise above the pain, but many people find a way to make the experience fruitful. There is often a desire to help others through their suffering. And one is never too young. For instance, a ten-year-old girl named Maria was taking a shower when an earthquake struck. The glass from the shower door broke, leaving cuts all over her body. She underwent multiple surgeries and painful treatments in addition to the grief of being called "a monster" by the boys in her school. Her parents brought her for EMDR therapy. During the last session she opened her eyes wide and exclaimed: *"Now I know why this happened to me. Because cut, burned and injured children will believe in me when I'll tell them that there is hope for them."*

The bottom line is that whatever the disability, people are able to reclaim themselves. I often think of the words of a dear colleague who has since passed away. Ron Martinez was a star athlete who prided himself on his body. One day he took a dive into a swimming pool, his neck twisted, and he had to be dragged back out. In one split second he became a quadriplegic. But he wouldn't quit. He became the first in his family to attend college and a therapist who was a shining light to those who knew him. His motto was "It's not what happens that matters. It's how you deal with it." We may not be responsible for the cause of our misery, but we can now take control and do something about it.

PERSONAL EXPLORATION

If you are suffering from any of the body issues described in this chapter, you can use the Floatback technique described in Chapter 4 to identify any memories that may be driving them. Concentrate on the feelings you have about the condition, and see if any of the negative cognitions from the three categories fit. If not, just notice the kinds of thoughts that come up when you focus on the last time you felt disturbance, and allow your mind to scan back to see if any memories emerge. If they do, put them on your *Touchstone List*.

As I said before, EMDR therapy will not eliminate a purely physical medical condition. But many of the feelings we have about ourselves when there is an actual illness or disability are caused by the unprocessed memories of careless remarks or our own feelings of wanting to be someone or something else. Many of us have had harsh parents, teachers or coaches who drummed unreasonable standards into us.

Many of us have forgotten the remarks consciously, but they are still there in our memory networks. It can actually be a good thing when children show obvious symptoms, because they are able to get the help they need immediately instead of quietly suffering for years.

For example, Britney is a bright, athletic, attractive 11-year-old. Her mother brought her in for treatment after she began pulling her eyelashes out. She'd started doing it at the beginning of the school year when her new, very critical teacher began yelling at the class. There were also other sources of stress, including her mother starting a new business and Britney feeling too upset to go to her much-loved gymnastics class because of her male coach's yelling. Initially during the EMDR treatment, the therapist targeted the first time the teacher yelled. That reduced the eyelash pulling to about one time a month, but didn't eliminate it. So they decided to target the coach's yelling. The therapist asked Britney to describe the worst part of the incident and her eyes opened wide as she said, "When he yelled and turned his back and said in a loud whisper, 'I'm going to kill you all. I'm going to kill you all with nails.'"

Sometimes, what children heard or saw can cause strong immediate symptoms, such as eyelash or hair pulling, or any of the symptoms that Bradley had. Or they can stay stored in memory networks and come up to bite years later. So as you try the Floatback, make sure to scan through memories of classmates, teachers, coaches, doctors, clergy—and any other important figure in your life. Britney's teacher and coach may have just thought they were doing their jobs. Maybe they didn't realize they could be scarring the children for life. Maybe they didn't care. Unfortunately, no matter what they thought—it doesn't matter. They may have caused damage, and now it's our job to repair it.

LIGHTSTREAM TECHNIQUE

For those of you with physical pain, the following is a guided imagery technique that may assist you. It can often help emotional pain disappear by at least temporarily helping you to change the way you are feeling. It can also help make physical pain more manageable. As with all the other self-control techniques, it's up to you to decide if it handles enough of the problem or if it would be a good idea to seek further assistance.

This technique is very useful for certain kinds of physical as well as emotional pain. It can also be helpful as a quick energy enhancer. It should be done in the comfort of your home or office. After you use it, give yourself a little time to relax before doing anything important. Read through the exercise until you memorize it and then follow the steps. If you have trouble with that, tape record your voice so it can lead you through the steps. There is also a prerecorded version available that you will see listed in Appendix A.

If you are feeling disturbed, concentrate on the upsetting body sensations. Identify the following by asking yourself: *"If it had a* _____, *what would it be?"* Fill in the blank with each word below.

a) shape

b) size

c) color

d) temperature

e) texture

f) sound (high pitched or low)

Just notice the shape and its other characteristics.

Now: *"What is your favorite color, or one you associate with healing?"*

Now imagine that a light of this color is coming in through the top of your head and directing itself at the shape in your body. Let's pretend that the source of this light is the cosmos, so you have an endless supply. **The light directs itself at the shape and resonates, vibrates in and around it. And as it does, what happens to the shape, size or color?**

If you find that the negative feelings change, then continue the Lightstream until you feel comfortable. If they don't change, then use your Safe/Calm Place arsenal, Spiral or breathing techniques to come back to neutral.

Clients have reported positive effects with the Lightstream technique for years. A recent study indicates that it may also prove to be useful for insomnia. In Indonesia, both the Safe Place and Lightstream techniques were used in combination to address sleep disturbance. Researchers reported the effects with five women who had been traumatized by receiving a diagnosis of HIV. They were all burdened by terrible feelings of fear, shame and insecurity because of their perception of the disease as horrible, along with the stigma in their culture that left them feeling dishonored. Their clinicians taught them the Safe Place in order to bring up feelings of comfort and relaxation. Then the Lightstream technique was directed at any negative body sensations. Within three days, all the women were able to sleep easily. Since that time an additional 106 people have been treated, and 75% have reported improved sleep. Those who didn't couldn't imagine a safe place. That included a number of people in prison—where life is very unsafe. While more research is necessary, this appears promising enough for me to suggest that you try it if you are having trouble sleeping. There are obviously no side effects, and we can all use help in this area occasionally.

CHAPTER
8

WHAT DO YOU WANT
FROM ME?

W hy is it that we often can't get along with family, friends or coworkers? "Blood is thicker than water, right? So why do I feel like strangling my brother?" "My wife just won't let up on me. It makes me want to run and hide." "We've been married for ten years, and he keeps doing things he knows make me crazy." *"How could he?" "How dare she?" "Why did they?"* Righteous indignation, anger, pain, guilt—mostly coming down to feeling wounded, misunderstood, discounted, unappreciated. See me! Respect my wants, my needs. It all seems reasonable. But it's a balancing act with different views, wounds and sometimes a bottomless pit of pain that shows up when you least expect it. Take the problems we've dealt with in previous chapters and multiply them by the number of people you run into on a typical day. It's not difficult to see that being in a relationship can stir up feelings that can be hard to deal with or understand.

WOUNDED NEEDS

No one is simple. We are all the product of an interaction between our genetic makeup and our experiences. Sometimes we can inherit predispositions to a variety of vulnerable states. Nevertheless, the majority of problems we might face are not due to our genetic makeup alone. In general, our sense of who we are and what we want from the world is governed by both processed and unprocessed memories. They underlie our conscious and unconscious responses. We have a hard enough time understanding ourselves. How are we supposed to understand anyone else? Many times we may need help. There are about 15 different kinds of family therapy and they assist people to understand the different patterns and problems in communication. For most family and couple therapists, there is the belief that if the way people interact with each other can be changed, then the relationships can become healthy and productive. Unfortunately, many times it's like trying to swim against a current, since the early childhood memories continue to drive unhealthy responses. People may want to change their actions but find themselves locked into patterns that they can't control. However, as we've already seen, understanding where our actions come from can be an important step in learning what we need to do to change.

What about Me?

Clinicians often think about relationships in terms of the attachment categories we covered in Chapter 5. When parents have an insecure attachment, they treat their children in certain ways. Then when these children grow up, they often fall into similar types of relationships with the same types of interactions. For instance, Alexandra came into therapy describing herself as depressed. She was 37 years old, twice divorced, and in an unhappy relationship with Joe for the past five years. She described him as someone "I can't live with and can't live without." They'd broken up numerous times but she kept going back to him.

Alexandra's primary complaint about Joe was that he either criticized her or ignored her. She was unable to speak up for herself even though she knew she "should," but always gave up, thinking to herself, "What's the use? It won't make a difference anyway." In her worst moments, Alexandra believed that she didn't deserve any better, as it had never been any different. Somehow, all of her relationships with men had turned out the same way. Although they always seemed to promise more in the beginning, she was left with trampled feelings and the sense that nothing was ever going to change.

Alexandra's history made everything she was going through easy to understand. As the youngest of four children, she was often criticized by her mother and ignored by her father. Her brothers bullied her and Alexandra would be blamed for their actions even though she did nothing to provoke them. She described coming home from school as early as the first grade with no one to greet her. Then she was punished for going to a neighbor's house to wait until her parents came home. The only one who seemed to love her was her grandfather and he died when she was six years old. Alexandra remembered feeling despair, sure that no one else would love her the way he did. No one seemed to care. For instance, at the age of eight, she was at a playground with her entire family when a bee stung her. Everyone ignored her and she remembered trying to "shove down" her pain, deciding "it didn't hurt." From that point on her feelings went underground, as she felt that her needs and her emotions were not important. After all, she "wasn't good enough" to get the love and attention her brothers received.

Alexandra's parents showed what is called a "dismissive" attachment style—being uncomfortable with closeness and strong emotions. Parents with this attachment style often withdraw and shy away from their children's feelings and needs. In turn, the lack of positive feelings and support generally lead their children to suppress their own feelings and desires for comfort. They are often left feeling not good enough and not worthy of attention. Alexandra couldn't express herself to Joe because his responses and those of her parents were so similar. Just as when she was a child, she was left feeling that she just wasn't important.

Concentrating on the last time Joe ignored her, a Floatback brought her back to the aloneness she felt in her family as a kid. Processing revealed multiple experiences where she was either criticized and rejected or neglected and ignored by her family, which paralleled her later relationships with men. Alexandra not only made bad romantic choices, but she also lacked the skills to identify and express her feelings and needs. Given the combination of childhood events, including the death of her grandfather, the feelings of unworthiness combined with loneliness and despair were triggered for Alexandra when she tried to end her relationships. There was a lot to process. Within the year, however, she left Joe for good. Now she was able to tolerate being alone without the desolation that had accompanied her early life.

As she began dating again, Alexandra noticed a different pattern emerging. Before, she remembered "losing herself" by trying to figure out what the other person wanted her to be and then becoming that person, hoping that she would be loved and accepted. Now Alexandra noticed that old pattern change, because she could "*feel herself.*" Being in touch with a sense of self-worth, it now made her feel bad to "give herself away." She started choosing men differently, breaking up with them without regret if they were not giving her what she needed. Her current partner is very supportive of her—including the ongoing challenges with her parents and her brothers, as she demands from them the respect she deserves as a loving and capable adult. While Alexandra needed help to learn new ways to communicate, she was no longer swimming against the current. Her childhood memories were no longer kicking up feelings of unworthiness and "nobody cares."

Useful Communication Skills

Some of the skills that Alexandra learned can be helpful to you if you have the same problem of not being in touch with your feelings or are unable to communicate them. For instance, before she left Joe, Alexandra and her clinician worked with a number of situations that generated some anxiety, to help her express her feelings to him. First, she needed help to get in touch with her emotions, so she concentrated on instances where he ignored her. Then she would examine: "If I were to have a feeling (right now), what would it be?" Or: "What would be the thoughts I would have?" Or: "What, then, would I say/do given my thinking about the situation?" The kinds of situations she explored included feeling that she would like to talk with him—instead of him watching a game on television. Or letting him know it made her uncomfortable for him to hang out in her living room for the evening without making an attempt to connect with her. With her clinician she developed a hierarchy of responses, ranging from the most gentle "This is how I'm feeling . . . I would like you to . . . " to the most insistent "If you're going to continue to behave this way, I need you to leave."

So if you aren't sure of what you feel, try to imagine what a trusted friend or someone you admire might feel in the same situation. Then how would you imagine that person communicating the feeling and desire? If your problem is the opposite—feeling too much—then try to observe your response, rather than be in it. Is this response useful? Will it serve me? It is also important to ask yourself, "Is my reaction coming from a child place or an adult place in me?" Sometimes the things we feel the need to express are coming from unprocessed emotions. That's the problem we'll explore in the next section.

Who Can I Blame?

Alexandra learned to accept unacceptable treatment from others in order to try to prevent feelings of rejection, aloneness and abandonment because her parents were rejecting and judgmental. In a similar situation, George learned something else entirely. He came to therapy extremely depressed because he couldn't seem to maintain a long-term relationship. The latest in a series of girlfriends had just broken up with him because he was too critical. If she was a little late getting ready to go out with him, he'd jump on her for being inconsiderate. If she cooked, the odds were he'd complain about something, like the meal wasn't hot enough. Basically, instead of complimenting her or showing his appreciation for what she did for him, he'd angrily complain about something that didn't please him. He wanted intimacy and love, but his automatic response was that something the other person was doing was wrong. Once again, the problem could be traced back to how his parents responded—not only to him, but also to each other.

George's parents had an extremely difficult life and came to this country as refugees from an oppressive regime. They often became anxious and overwhelmed because of their own triggers, resulting in a "preoccupied" attachment style. Dealing with their own pain, they were often unable to notice what their children required. For their own survival, children with these types of parents often use anger, temper tantrums and vocal demands to get their needs met. Not surprisingly, George wasn't close with his siblings, since they grew up competing for their parents' attention. They would argue and fight frequently. Add to this the fact that George's father was extremely critical of his mother and had a "very short fuse"—showing a lot of anger when around the house—and you have the perfect model for George's current behavior. Just as his father acted with his mother and with him, nothing was ever good enough and he automatically made it known.

While we all have desires and preferred ways of doing things, it's good to evaluate whether we are being thoughtful or having a "knee-jerk" reaction. How much heat goes along with our response? Are we even observing how our words are affecting the other person? Is it coming from an adult place or not? The types of chronic critical responses George had can often be traced back to specific childhood experiences that get triggered in relationships. Looking back, he remembered many examples of his father's anger and criticism, and of his mother being very judgmental. For his mother, nothing was good enough either. While he described his mother as manipulative and demanding, his father was more oppressive. He had no hesitation in humiliating his wife or children for their supposed shortcomings. George remembered his father as constantly yelling at him for doing something wrong—starting with not picking up his toys or making too much noise when he was four years old. Over time, George developed the sense of being defective and in danger, verbalized by the negative beliefs: "I'm not good enough," "I'm not safe" and "I can't trust other people." So whenever a girlfriend didn't meet his needs, it triggered his old feelings and produced the kind of angry, critical responses he'd witnessed between his father and mother. Not exactly the kind of interactions most women are looking for in a healthy relationship.

Generally, the reason that women have for putting up with this type of behavior for any length of time is that they have childhoods similar to Alexandra's, where they are used to not getting their own needs met.

Ultimately, the goal is for both partners to react to each other from a healthy adult perspective, not from the perspective colored by childhood pain. Just as Alexandra was liberated from her destructive pattern by processing her earlier memories, so was George. A pivotal change for him came through letting go of his anger at his parents as he recognized their limitations—and how their own history had caused them to behave in those ways. Draining the pool of anger he had carried since childhood, along with his own feeling of being defective, allowed him to be more present in his relationships as an adult, not as a wounded child.

FILLING THE VOID

Anisha is a 21-year-old woman from India who now, after successful therapy, wishes to share her story. It can help shed light on what it feels like to be "blinded in love"—grasping onto the wrong person to fill needs that should be met in other ways. Anisha had always been a trusting child, eager to please. But when she was 17 years old, her world seemed to fall apart. As she describes it:

My uncle lost his temper in a minor dispute and unleashed his rage by beating me relentlessly. My father was present but did not come to my aid. I was shattered. I felt broken, and the security I'd felt with my family was lost. I was joyless, and my relationship with my parents and extended family deteriorated.

This pushed her into the arms of Gorakh, a young man she had met a couple of years before. It was not a partnership of equals. He became everything to her. *I tried to put my feelings about my family in the past and move forward. I had Gorakh. I had a chance at happiness. I came to believe that it was only Gorakh I could love. That he was someone I could pin all my hopes and desires on. I loved him solely for who he was, or at least the idea that I built in my head. I gave more than myself to our relationship. But what I realized much too late was that Gorakh clearly reveled in the fact that I put him on a pedestal and accommodated my life to suit his needs. I ran every errand, bathed his dog, did everything he asked of me. Anything at all to please him. Unfortunately, it didn't seem to be enough and when the novelty wore off, he abruptly carved me away like a rotten piece of fruit. But my love for him didn't die. No amount of his constant neglect and arrogance changed anything. I saw him always as the love of my life. Whenever it suited him, he enjoyed having me around. I was the one person who loved him no matter what. Then I became pregnant and Gorakh abandoned me. He wanted to have nothing to do with me. From then on I was only a burden he was desperate to shake off.*

All I remember after is the reality of the sonogram confirming I was pregnant, my mother's shock and hurt, my father's cold disappointment, and the agonizing guilt of having to terminate my pregnancy. I remember waking up mornings with my wrists sliced open almost to the bone, my pillowcases soaked in blood and tears, and the constant pain in my chest and lungs that wouldn't let me breathe—like there was a void. I'd lost everything. Everything was meaningless.

Once again, the message is that regardless of the amount of pain—or how desperate the situation seems to be—it is the unprocessed memories that are running the show. Anisha now feels very different. As she puts it: *Over the eight months of therapy, I felt myself gradually transform into a more neutral and rational human being. Now I feel like a new person. For this I'm eternally grateful.* If you feel stuck in a bed of pain, either because of desperately clinging to a person who doesn't value you, or because of feeling used and abandoned, you can choose a new pathway. We all deserve relationships that give us joy and that support our self-worth. If you aren't feeling that, then consider what is keeping you stuck. As you learn new ways to cope and the unprocessed memories are transformed—you can be too.

THE DANCE OF DESTRUCTION

When we hear stories of domestic abuse, many of us are puzzled about how these types of experiences happen. "How could he act that way?" "Why did she let it happen?" The answer is generally that it is simply a more extreme example of the kinds of memories that can get locked into the brain and the ways they push our thoughts, emotions and behaviors. There is a wide variety of destructive couples' interactions that can range from ongoing verbal conflicts to physical abuse. Some conflicts can be worked out together between the couple. But sometimes the abuse becomes a cycle that all the agreements in the world won't stop. In those cases, the work needs to be done individually with therapeutic assistance. Couples therapy is not a first choice, or even a good choice, for most abusive couples. It is important to remember that "verbal violence," which involves being intimidated, threatened, belittled or humiliated, can also have devastating emotional effects. It has even been found to contribute substantially to postpartum depression. Violence, verbal or physical, is an individual issue. Each partner needs separate treatment first. Then, if there are still "couples" issues, a qualified therapist can be consulted. A list of resources is available in Appendix B.

It's easy for some people with these kinds of destructive relationship patterns to look fine when dating or prior to intimacy—in fact, that is how they partner up to begin with. It's often not until people are in a committed relationship or even living together that the problems begin.

For others, where a partner has a history of being controlling, the domination often starts when dating. However, as with Anisha, for many couples the glaze of new love seems to cover up the true meaning of the controlling behavior. The problems really heat up as the intimacy grows and the old triggers start to get hit more often. In most cases it is the unhealed pain from the past that is often triggering the current reactions in this new "family" situation.

The way in which people respond to emotional pain varies because of their trauma histories and the environments they were brought up in. This includes the kinds of interactions they saw in the childhood home. For instance, the feelings of "I'm not good enough/I'm worthless" can result in anger and lashing out, or submission and collapse because "nobody cares." Sometimes it escalates to levels of ongoing verbal or physical abuse. The person who is being abused reacts to the threat and pain of the current situation. Yet people may remain in that kind of relationship because of their own trauma history.

Of course, there are exceptions. Some people get trapped in ongoing unhealthy relationships due to financial hardship, cultural expectation or extreme forms of control. But our goal here is to explore the psychological dynamics that are common in these kinds of interactions. They happen more often than you may think and may be affecting you or people around you. In the next section, we'll look at couples in conflict at the level of verbal abuse. In general, the major question is: How long will either of the partners wait before insisting on change?

Anger Mismanagement

Jack was referred into treatment because his wife's therapist had asked him to come in for one couple's session. The clinician asked some questions and saw a connection between his current behavior and his past. She referred him for EMDR therapy since she was concerned about his combative and controlling behaviors and his history of trauma. He and Mary had been together for three years. While he'd never directly assaulted her, he had damaged her personal property, and their arguments had become more frequent and volatile. These are warning signs that further abuse may be about to happen. Mary had recently set a limit with him—he needed to attend individual therapy and change his actions, or he would have to move out of their apartment. Through her own EMDR therapy, she had dealt with her own childhood issues. She was now capable of leaving the relationship, was financially independent and was planning to do just that if he didn't change.

Jack had tried therapy before, but it hadn't worked for him. This isn't surprising, since the feelings from childhood that prevent healthy adult relationships can also exist in the therapist's office. Happily, Jack arrived at the office of a very skilled clinician who was adept at treating these issues. Nevertheless, during the first sessions he resisted looking inward and focused instead on stories to highlight Mary's many "flaws"—none of which seemed valid—while avoiding his therapist's attempts to gather a thorough history. He missed several of their first appointments and showed up late to others. In the sessions he did attend, he described a pattern of current alcohol and marijuana abuse, depressive symptoms and a suicide attempt at age 21 after a relationship ended abruptly. Basically, he was a human being in pain who was now inflicting emotional distress on Mary.

His current mental state and the fact that his behavior was nudging Mary out of the picture raised additional concerns. So his therapist met with both of them to create a clear plan: to prevent escalation into physical violence. Mary needed a plan to keep herself safe if Jack got abusive.

Jack needed a plan to stop his behavior for her sake and for his. His actions were only increasing his sense of failure, which fed the negative cycle. Jack was asked to notice when he felt triggered into anger—and then to put the issues "on hold" and "walk away" instead of taking it up with Mary. He was encouraged to bring the "issues" to therapy in order to develop a more productive response. He initially resisted, but after discussing it further, he admitted that "his way" wasn't working.

Mary agreed to leave temporarily if Jack appeared triggered and seemed unable to "walk away." Jack had no history of stopping Mary from leaving if she wanted to, and he indicated no hesitation about either of them leaving if needed. This constituted a workable short-term plan. The fact that Mary had already decided (and both therapists agreed) that he would need to move out immediately if he did not follow the plan— and eventually if change did not occur soon—helped to increase his motivation. While not thrilled with having to attend therapy, he was sincere about saving his relationship and agreed to try a new way.

At the next session, Jack eagerly agreed to provide his therapist with the "play by play" on his recent angry thoughts about Mary, particularly his distress over behaviors and choices she had made before they had ever met. During these discussions it was easy to see the insecurity, fear of failure, shame, a deep sense of inadequacy and powerlessness behind the anger. Jack struggled to understand and address the issues along with his actions that he didn't fully believe were wrong. He would rant in fury toward Mary and a few moments later tearfully express his fear about losing one of the best relationships he ever had. He agreed to give EMDR processing a try.

During the next session, Jack began by complaining about a recent fight with Mary. His therapist noticed that while discussing the fight he placed his hands on his chest. They did a Floatback from that sensation and found their first target, a memory of an angry fight between his parents when he was ten years old, one of many battles in the war at home that never resolved. It was the first time he could see and feel the connection between his past and present. His negative cognition was "I am powerless." His choice for a positive cognition was "I have choices now." Many things now began to make sense.

It took several sessions to completely reprocess this particular memory, but at each reevaluation Jack and his therapist could see that the work was paying off. His insight increased dramatically along with his compassion for both himself and Mary. As he processed the fighting he had witnessed as a child, the urges to provoke arguments in his present home decreased. For the first time, he could openly discuss how powerless he had felt as he watched the two people he loved the most destroy each other and how that had impacted his ability to see relationships as anything but a war zone—places of unending pain and struggle, where issues could never be resolved. Lastly, he started to digest a painful reality—his current behavior, particularly his jealousy about Mary's past, closely mimicked that of his abusive father.

After completing the reprocessing of that initial target, Jack worked on other memories related to his feeling of powerlessness. He stopped drinking and drugging, started working out at the local gym, and kept a calm, open dialogue going with Mary, who continued working with her own EMDR therapist to address her own issues. Jack and his therapist continued to monitor his reactions for emotional upheavals, but he no longer felt triggered in the same way. He told his therapist that while he could be angry and frustrated at times, something had really changed inside of him. He demonstrated by putting his hands on his chest, as he had done during that initial Floatback, and said: "I don't have that feeling anymore. I've had that feeling for as long as I can remember, but it just isn't there anymore."

After their EMDR memory processing was completed, Jack and Mary were referred to couples therapy with the focus on building relationship skills, since neither had learned as children how to deal with disagreements while maintaining a connection to each other. Both admitted that their parents simply had not possessed these skills. They, on the other hand, felt they could learn them and wanted to teach them to the children they planned to have in the future. Far from feeling "I am powerless," now Jack's behaviors indicate that he is a man who believes he can be an agent for positive change in his life and in the life of the family he is starting.

At his initial session, Jack's therapist had asked him to write down his reason for coming to therapy. He had written: "I want to get over the past." In clarifying this, he'd told his therapist that he wanted to get over Mary's past. He didn't think he had a past that he needed to work on. He simply thought he had to find a way to deal with *her* past. Happily, he achieved that goal, although not quite in the way he had anticipated.

Useful Relationship Skills

Some of the skills that Jack and Mary learned from their respective therapists can be useful additions to any relationship. It's important to think of interactions on a continuum. While Jack and Mary's relationship was becoming increasingly dangerous as the anger and arguments escalated, all of us experience times when we get triggered and angry. Sometimes it gets to the point where we are taking our own stuff out on our partners. I'll include a section at the end of this chapter with more skills that can be useful, but here are a few that most directly pertain to relationships involving anger.

Create a plan—a firm agreement between you and your partner about how to manage escalating anger to protect both of you from hurting each other and to protect any children from witnessing the arguments. Parental arguments can have devastating effects on children and shatter their sense of safety. The agreement can include a "Time-Out" plan. It involves telling your partner that you need a "Time-Out" and both of you deciding when to come back and discuss the issue in a nonemotional manner. If you don't see immediate results from sticking to the plan, consult a therapist or a local domestic violence program for professional assistance. Agreements only work if both parties can actually commit to and follow them. For some couples this is simply not possible without professional intervention from a qualified domestic violence therapist. For others, even outside assistance will not be sufficient. Know when "enough is enough."

Look for the trends—don't get too caught up in the content. Try to puzzle out the pattern of your fighting—perhaps notice when it typically happens, where it happens, the theme of what you fight about, and the ways it does/doesn't resolve. During a neutral/nonangry time, discuss the themes and try to work on them together, agreeing to take a Time-Out or seek a neutral helper to assist if you get stuck. Try to take the stance that it is the two of you looking at the problem together—as a team.

Know your own "triggers"—issues or scenarios that ignite strong emotions or unproductive reactions. Educate your partner about these and agree upon a way to inform your partner that you're triggered so you can disengage from interacting until you feel calmer. Educate yourself about your partner's triggers also. This will help increase your insight into, and therefore compassion for, the issues that have created these triggers for both of you. Role-play with each other how you would like your partner to respond to you.

Push You, Pull Me

While most of us have a variety of wounds from childhood, some of us have lived through experiences that seem more like nightmares. Linda fell into that category—and it affected both her own happiness and her relationships. When she was just a baby, her mother had given her away to a relative in order to pursue a dancing career. Then two years later she returned and demanded Linda back, which resulted in the toddler literally being taken away screaming from the arms of the only parents she had ever known. Linda was then verbally and physically abused throughout her childhood by her alcoholic mother, who made the child feel that she was a terrible person. In addition, Linda was molested by her stepfather when she was very young, and then by a female cousin when she was ten years old. When she told her mother about it, she was made to feel that it was all her fault. Her teenage years were filled with bullying and humiliations at home and at school—and becoming an adult brought little relief. After seven years of marriage, she found out that her husband, the person she believed was her soul mate, was having an affair with one of her relatives. Then later she discovered that her 15-year-old cousin had molested her 3-year-old son and her young daughter.

At the age of 43 she came into therapy with low self-esteem, depression, anxiety and severe marital problems. The chaos created by her pathological jealousy, temper tantrums and the rage attacks that she directed at her husband, Leonard, became too much for him to bear. He finally threatened to divorce her if something didn't change. She had been in therapy for two years previously and had gained insight about her past—but her reactions hadn't changed. Leonard had taken responsibility for his behavior, was fully committed to their marriage and showed it in every way possible. Linda knew this intellectually, but her emotional responses were fed by all her earlier trauma.

When people have been as badly abused as Linda, all of their relationships can suffer. Many of us have relatives, acquaintances, coworkers that we just don't understand. Why do they keep acting like children? The failed relationships of all kinds—marriages, friendships, stepparents, in-laws or coworkers—are often a product of the volcano of emotions that are stored in the unprocessed memory networks. Sometimes nice, other times insensitive or raging—these people are often triggered in ways that are hard to understand. Add to that the fact that they never learned self-soothing skills as children, as well as the difficulties they have feeling empathy for others since they never received it from their parents. It's not hard to see why life often becomes one set of personality clashes after another. Anxiety, depression, suicide attempts are often part of the picture—as deep down inside there are unprocessed memory networks that cause them to feel terrified and of no importance.

After processing all the traumas, including the infidelity, Linda and Leonard are now happily married and want to share their experience in the hope of helping others. So here is their message in order to offer some insight for couples in their situation, or for those who are looking on hopelessly, trying to deal with someone who seems out of control. According to Linda:

We were in a repetitive pattern of dysfunction. I was extremely sensitive to anything that sounded like abandonment, including being ignored by my husband or him walking away when I was talking. I would lose it if he walked away. It was bizarre—even I didn't understand it! We really didn't know how to communicate. Neither one of us was listening to the other. I cried a lot, sometimes over things that seemed important, other times I just felt like crying.

There was a sense of having to have drama in my life, which was a product of my childhood, living with an alcoholic mom. I would have unrealistic expectations and would often sabotage our good times together—or if we went too long without an argument, I would find a way to start one. I needed that stimulus, good or bad. I was quick to anger and had very little patience. This was a button for him. I would get frustrated when trying to get a point across and he would shut down the minute I got angry. I didn't feel like he valued me, and he felt like I didn't respect him. I didn't like being alone and always questioned him about his whereabouts. Of course this infuriated him, and he would go off on me.

After EMDR, what really blew my mind was that I discovered who I really am. I enjoyed being alone. I looked forward to that time. I wasn't as scared or insecure anymore. I had a new sense of self. I was able to identify what I wanted, and I went after it. Also, I was more trusting. The arguments went way down. We learned how to compromise without feeling like we were giving up something. I learned to love in a different way. I found I got more out of the relationship than before. I asked for what I wanted rather than expecting him to know what I wanted.

My advice for other couples is to really evaluate how much your relationship is worth and how much you have invested. Don't be hasty to call it quits. If you really love each other—do the work. It's easy to walk away, but what will you have learned? How will you prevent repeating the same mistakes again with another person? There's a reason people who divorce have multiple marriages. There may be underlying issues from the past that are getting in the way of your ability to love, trust, respect.

Having heated arguments doesn't mean the marriage is destined to fail. Here is Leonard's view on how appropriate help can turn things around:

Before therapy, I was alternately flattered and thrilled or mystified and angry. On the one hand, Linda was a skilled, generous and imaginative woman. But on the other hand, she could be very arbitrary, with mood swings that left me in the dust. I was at a loss to justify the difference between these two personalities.

We each learned that there are more effective ways of resolving marriage conflicts than through emotion. You can replace pointless, emotion-based bickering with thoughtful, result-oriented resolutions to differences that arise in the course of forging a lasting, loving and bonding relationship. The big difference before/after EMDR was really trust. After EMDR there was a solid, unchanging foundation to our relationship. Once that new dynamic was established, there followed many years of trust building like we had never had before. We used our new foundation to bring real, time-tested strength to our marriage.

As you can see, Linda and Leonard communicate in very different ways. Linda had often felt discounted, thinking Leonard didn't value her emotions. Leonard had felt the same way, believing that Linda didn't value his logic. As with many couples, their relationship strengthened as they became able to communicate without getting their buttons pushed. As Leonard put it, "We learned that a successful marriage needs passion, emotion AND intellect, but all in the appropriate time and place." For any couple, life gets easier when unprocessed memories aren't in the way.

What's Getting Triggered?

It's important to remember that sometimes the current situation can be triggering something completely unsuspected and seemingly unrelated. One example is Ava, who also couldn't sustain a healthy romantic relationship. She was raised by a single mom who was an active drug addict. In addition, one of her mother's long-term boyfriends was both sadistic and sexually abusive to Ava throughout her early teens. While Ava made reasonably good choices with female friendships, all of her past relationships with men had been sexually, physically and emotionally abusive. She was currently involved in an "on and off" relationship with Oscar. While he wasn't physically or sexually abusive, he had a history of becoming verbally abusive and frequently abandoned her with little warning. As a couple, they struggled with explosive arguments—which often ended with Ava pulling out her own hair in frustration. Processing a number of her early memories, including those of her mother's abusive boyfriend, resulted in her feeling much better about herself, but didn't change the relationship pattern. So, after a comprehensive assessment of the situation, Oscar was asked to come in for a joint session.

Oscar described Ava as calm, supportive, independent and sweet, yet also jealous, angry and controlling. Ava described Oscar as a "good man" who she felt committed to, but also noted that she feared his tendency to flee the relationship when "things got tough." She discussed feeling "out of control" when upset with Oscar, which triggered him to "run" from the relationship because of his fear of escalating violence—something he had witnessed often as a child. He was also put off by her "paranoid jealousy and rage" when it came to his friendships with other women.

The therapist asked Ava's permission to do a Floatback with Oscar present, starting with the "out of control" feeling she experienced in a recent fight. The technique landed her at nine years old in her living room, screaming at her mother to stay home and not leave her alone for the evening. In the memory Ava punched the walls until her fists bled in an attempt to capture her mother's attention and avoid abandonment because of her mother's preoccupation with her own relationship. The problem was really feeling "I'm unimportant" and fear of being left alone. Oscar and Ava left that session more understanding of the pain their fighting triggered. Ava had also unearthed her next EMDR target. Processing that childhood memory changed the relationship dynamic. She was able to communicate her needs and desires without fear or drama.

Another Relationship Tip

Don't be embarrassed to ask for help. TV programs often show the joys and sorrows of finding love, yet never stick around to explain or highlight all the difficult parts of working it out. If you didn't learn how to be in a relationship growing up, perhaps you may need to read a book, attend a class or see a therapist for assistance. This is not inborn stuff. We are supposed to learn this from our parents, but they can't teach us what they did not know themselves. Yet, for the sake of our children and the others we love, we do need to learn it. The bottom line is that for a healthy adult relationship, there need to be two emotionally healthy adults.

TO HAVE OR HAVE NOT

We often hear people say that although they are searching, they can't seem to find anyone who is interested in a committed relationship. Others say that while marriage might be fine for others, they simply "don't believe in it." When questioned, they might talk about how unhappy their parents were together, and that they don't want to lock themselves into that kind of prison. Others who have lived through the grief of their parents' divorce don't want to take the chance. Unfortunately, they believe that history is bound to repeat itself. While that is likely if history is left unattended, it doesn't have to be true. We can learn from our parents' mistakes—and also undo the damage that was done growing up in pain. Even if we've had previous relationships that didn't work, we can learn from our own mistakes and make better choices.

Freedom to Choose

As we've seen, there are reasons for current relationship problems. There can be early childhood fears that are locked into our memory networks that we may or may not be aware of. We can also get caught in destructive patterns that cause us to choose the wrong partners. Many of these patterns are caused by relationships with our parents that are based on *their* maladaptive solutions that we simply could not avoid. For instance, we can be run by the emotional baggage handed off to us by our parents because we were caught in what many family therapists call "triangles"— a way of relating with our parents that helped them cope with their problems. Sometimes when there is stress in a marriage, the parents focus on a "special child" to relieve the pressure. Whether the child is "special" because of accomplishment or need, they can become the center of attention. Other times, when there is marital conflict, a parent will choose one of the children to be his or her "special child." That was the case with Sonia.

Sonia came from a working class Italian family. She initially came in to therapy because of depression, feelings of hopelessness and lack of meaning in her life. She had never been married, unlike her two sisters who both had husbands and children. At 34 years old, she saw herself as the odd one in a family that put a high value on raising kids. She was lonely and socially isolated, and never seemed to find men who could nurture and support her.

Her failures in finding love came from a childhood "triangle" where she was used by her father as a "favorite" to meet his own needs for emotional closeness. The family story was that Dad had a very abusive childhood. This was used to explain why he had such a bad temper. That was the "excuse" for slapping, swearing or raging at Sonia and his other children when they "misbehaved." However, as his special child, Sonia was the only one in the family who would confront or comfort him. Because of that, her mother resented her and often gave her the cold shoulder. Rather than go to his wife for appropriate emotional support, Sonia's father often used her to confide in about how tough his wife could be. Sonia then learned to seek out special attention from her father and share his negative view of her "impossible" mother. This was not hard to do, given her mother's negative attitude— and jealousy—toward her.

This triangle between Sonia and her two parents set her up for seeking out men who were not really available for emotional closeness and intimacy. It caused her to easily buy into an unavailable man's claim that his current wife or girlfriend was flawed, but that he was obligated to stay with her. It also primed her to accept emotional explosiveness in a partner who was exempt from responsibility because of his "difficult past." Early on, Sonia began to "settle" for boys who would fool around with her, but not really value her or offer her the legitimate status of being their girlfriend. Her relationship history was full of painful triangles and emotionally abusive men who "needed" her, but were not really able to be there for her in any kind of sustained way. Processing the painful memories with the encoded beliefs "I'm bad," "I'm unlovable" and "I don't deserve to be loved" liberated Sonia on many levels. Now she recognizes the danger signals and is choosing men who are also free to choose her. She's no longer interested in being the "other woman."

Holding Closed

For most of us, there is a desire for true intimacy with our loved one. We want to be able to share without any sense of danger, to be held and comforted when we need it, to laugh, to play and to be transported by passion with no fear of judgment. Unfortunately, for many people there has been little true intimacy, and for others it vanishes over time. In most cases, it's because something has disrupted the ability to trust. The lack of emotional safety keeps us from sharing our pain because we are afraid of how our partner will respond.

As we have seen, some of us have longstanding fears that prevent us from being close with a loved one. For instance, Emily was married to a man she truly loved. But for some reason that she couldn't understand, she was afraid that if she let down her guard, expressed herself and was really present with him, he would "disappear." She was aware of feeling shame, sadness and fear. The beliefs that went along with these feelings were "I'm unworthy," "I'm unimportant" and "I can't trust anyone." The feelings turned out to be grounded in two events in childhood: one where her mother forgot to pick her up from school when she was six years old. The second had happened at eight years old, when she and her family were at an amusement park. She had a tantrum and they got in the car and left her there. Now, obviously in both instances Emily's family eventually came back for her. But the damage was already done because the pain and fear she experienced were already locked into her memory network, setting the groundwork for her future relationships.

Emily's story is not an isolated case. As we examine where we are feeling unfulfilled or blocked in our relationships, we need to ask ourselves: What is preventing us from working with our partner as a team to solve our issues? Have we tried unsuccessfully to communicate? Or have we held back expressing ourselves? Very often, the inability to communicate our desires can be based on fears of expressing anger, being rejected or hearing an angry response. For others, it involves fear of saying, "No." Is it justified? Have you tried before and gotten emotionally smacked down in your current relationship? If not, it would be useful to use the Floatback technique to see if you can find a Touchstone Memory to explain your reaction, and use the Spiral, Lightstream or other techniques to shift it.

If you do find that you are being run by old stuff, try using the Safe Place exercise to give you the courage to express yourself. Let your partner know that expressing yourself is difficult and why. Explain that you'd like to work on the problem as a team. Consider professional assistance to help you. Unfortunately, many people think their partner should "just know" how they are feeling and what to do about it. It would be nice if we were all mind readers—but it doesn't work that way. When we have unexpressed needs that aren't being met, the feelings of being unimportant and "not good enough" are often part of our own unprocessed memory network of earlier experiences. It's now our responsibility to do something about it. Remember, it's "To have and to hold"—not withhold.

Where Did You Go?

As we've seen, some people choose relationships where no closeness is possible from the beginning. For others, something happens along the way. We close off—often leaving our partner confused, angry and in pain. What happened? Why is the relationship different? Where is the person I married? In these cases, self-doubt often creeps into the relationship. Sometimes the problems are caused by physical disability where one begins to feel like a burden, or financial problems where someone who was in the role of breadwinner feels like a failure. Power balances change through retirement or empty nests. Sometimes an accident or other trauma kicks up feelings of shame and guilt. These are times for a couple to come closer together. But sometimes the situation is so disturbing that something blocks that from happening. That was the case with Bart and Cindy. What started off as a true romance almost ended because of walls neither one knew how to take apart. They agreed to a posttreatment interview because they want to help other people in their position.

Bart and Cindy had been married for more than 15 years when they came into therapy. During their courtship and early marriage they had played, laughed and formed deep emotional and sexual bonds. But the past ten years, since Bart had returned from Operation Desert Storm, had been an emotional wasteland. As Cindy put it:

We got farther and farther apart. I mean I tried really, really hard to pretend things were OK, 'cause I couldn't find specifically what was wrong. Why were we unhappy? Why weren't we close? What was the problem? I couldn't figure it out. I had no clue. So our intimate relationship started feeling to me more like Bart was using the "high" he would get off of sex as a drug to escape whatever was giving him pain and make him feel worthwhile as a human being, but it wasn't about us loving each other. I mean that's the way it started to feel to me and I kept with it, trying to believe that we still had a marriage going on in this sexual relationship. But I was feeling abandoned and I was mad at him for it.

Bart had been deployed as a medic and never expected to pick up a gun. But during an ambush he'd been forced to kill a man, and it left him feeling guilty and ashamed. He was so devastated with guilt that he couldn't tell Cindy—as he was afraid she'd turn away from him completely. Cindy is the one who pushed for treatment because Bart no longer seemed to be the person she had married. He was no longer emotionally available to her—and this fractured their trust. For instance, he was so preoccupied with his own pain and so triggered by anything having to do with death, that when Cindy broke down after her father died, Bart ordered her to stop, saying, "One day of crying is enough."

But Bart was also afraid of losing her. So, feeling like a bad person, he became submissive and did everything he could to win her approval, including working overtime. Whenever she complained, he couldn't stand up for himself anymore because, as he put it, *I was a horrible person because of what I had done. And it was totally subconscious, I mean, there was just a feeling like I don't deserve to be happy, I don't deserve rewards from life. I deserve to make amends.* However, we are complex beings. Because Bart also felt resentful at Cindy's continued criticism, he'd be irritable in other ways. The pattern of emotional distance and discord was pushing them further and further away from each other. As she said, *The emptiness got bigger and bigger and bigger and bigger.*

Happily, through couples work and EMDR therapy, things are now back to normal—with both Bart and Cindy feeling as equals again. The advice that they have for war veteran couples holds true for all couples who find themselves blocked off and pushed further and further apart. Whatever you feel ashamed or guilty about, don't let it separate you from the ones you love. Your perspective about it now may simply be the unprocessed emotions that are keeping you locked up. For instance, according to Bart:

Before, I'd say to myself, "You are a horrible person. You should be ashamed of what you've done and you need to make up for it." Now it's, "I was put in a horrible situation, very unfortunate, but I did what I was instructed to do, which is what I agreed to do in the first place. You know, it's a life or death choice, and you accept the consequences that go with those. It's still a horrible tragedy that he had to die, and I still feel bad about that, but I don't think that I'm a bad person for what I did. . . . Get good intervention early, the sooner, the better—so there's not that much "baggage" that's stacked up on top. Cindy and I went through ten years before we got to this point. There's a lot of healing now that has to happen.

For Cindy, things are different as well. As she says, appearances can also be deceiving. But when you are closed off from your partner, your helpmate, your love—the pain is very real: *Bart was functioning perfectly, earning money, being a good father, paying bills, doing everything you're supposed to do. Not hitting anybody, not getting drunk, not going to jail, not doing anything bad. So how does anybody know his self-esteem is mortally wounded? And the veteran who might have had the war experience isn't the only person that might need EMDR therapy. I had some very strong emotional issues that I had to overcome too as a result of what occurred between us over time due to this experience that Bart had. So I would recommend getting both people involved in that kind of therapy.*

The results are worth the effort. As she describes it, after ten years of secret pain and of feeling isolated and used during sex, they are truly intimate again: *Now I feel like there is actual love for each other going on. If you look at it emotionally, it's black and white. I mean it is so totally different now than it has been in the past because I feel loved and appreciated. And so it is wonderful.*

The bottom line here is that if something happens that changes your relationship, be willing to communicate about it. If you find yourself blocked, try using the self-control techniques to change the way you feel. If that doesn't work, consider getting professional assistance. Waiting for things to blow over is not something that should be dragging on for months and years. As Bart said, it only adds to the "baggage."

YOU'RE BAD, I'M MAD

For all of us, there are times when we get hooked by a situation at work, with friends or with family. We strongly believe that some person is demonstrating bad behavior. We may be completely right, but are we really dealing with it appropriately? If we are overreacting because the situation is linking into some of our own unprocessed memories, it's simply not healthy for us. The stress can wear us down. For instance, Elena came from a close extended family that regularly got together, but her cousin Patrick often did not keep his word. If they were supposed to meet, he often arrived an hour late. If he agreed to call or do something, it rarely happened without repeated promptings. Elena continually found herself being triggered by her cousin. She'd told Patrick repeatedly that she believed that keeping one's word was important. If he said that he would do something, he should do it. If he couldn't do it on time, he should please let her know. That seemed very simple, but it did no good. Patrick would promise and then repeat the same actions.

As they say, you can pick your friends, but you can't pick your family. Elena rarely encountered this kind of behavior in others, because we choose to be friends with people who give us a certain comfort level. If any acquaintance had acted as Patrick did, Elena would not have bothered to continue the relationship. But Elena was stuck with her cousin and there were times she needed to interact with him because of family commitments. So the important thing at that point was to examine the amount of disturbance she felt.

Most of us would say that Patrick's behavior was unacceptable in an adult—but did that justify the intensity of Elena's emotional reaction? In other words, how much did it bother her, and was there anything she could do about it? We've all been in situations where people we've confided in have agreed that we were being subjected to inappropriate behavior, but they said we "shouldn't take it personally." If we understand that overreacting and "taking it personally" generally means that the situation is hooking into unprocessed memories, we can explore where our high level of emotions is coming from.

Elena concentrated on the last time Patrick had promised to do something and failed to keep his word. The thoughts that came to her mind were tinged with anger and resentment: "I always keep my word to him. Think of all the things I've done for him!" Then she asked herself: "How does that make me feel?" The answer was, "I'm not important enough for him to make the effort." The shorthand for that was feeling clearly, "I'm not important." So holding in mind the image of the last time Patrick had broken his word, and the thought "I'm not important," Elena used the Floatback technique and let her mind go back to the earliest memory she had when she felt that way. What came up was an image of herself as an adolescent. She and her friends had agreed to meet at a train stop to go into the city for the day. Elena waited past the appointed hour. She thought she saw them on a passing train, but no one got off at her stop. She trudged home disappointed and hurt. A little while later they called to say they'd been tied up fixing someone's hair and makeup. Since they hadn't expected her to wait for them, they had gone into the city without her. Now they were calling to see if she wanted to meet them. She joined them, but with the feeling of not having been important enough to really care about. That was what was being triggered by Patrick's behavior.

That realization was enough to allow her to see more clearly that her cousin behaved the same way with everyone in the family. He was constantly late and often forgot his commitments. Although Elena wasn't happy with Patrick's behavior, she was able to use the Breathing Shift and Spiral techniques to deal with her feelings when they came up, since she was no longer caught up in the righteous indignation. There was nothing she could do to change her cousin. All she could do was try to minimize the times she needed him to do something.

We can't pick our family. We often can't change them. But we can recognize when we are likely to be triggered and deal with our negative emotions and physical responses rather than buy into them with thoughts of "How dare he!" or "How could she!" Sometimes it helps to view the situation as an opportunity for our own personal exploration and growth. Elena recognized that the early memory of being left at the station had also influenced her choice of friends and colleagues. She had cut more than a few people out of her life who had failed to keep their word even once. Maybe it was time to give others a little more slack. She also decided to call her old therapist to process the memory—and any others that might be related. It's a good reminder for all of us when we get really upset. Whether it's with family, friends or coworkers, it's important to ask: Is this reaction coming from an adult or child place?

Clearly it's important to reduce stress in your life. For instance, continuing to be angry or upset by someone's behavior, especially when that person's actions have not really harmed you, may be pushed by your own power and control issues. You may be primarily upset that the person doesn't act as you'd like them to, and that you're powerless to change them. Although sometimes difficult, it's important to remember that the power to choose how others act is theirs. And your choices are about you. Try using your Safe/Calm Place and then quietly bring to mind the person who is bothering you and think the words, "I forgive you for being who you are." Do it a few times. You may find that after doing that, whenever you think of them, you won't be as upset. You may not like their actions, but continued resentment harms you more than it does them.

SOME FINAL RELATIONSHIP RECOMMENDATIONS

Look for the cause. Sometimes our pain over a family member's actions is compounded by feelings of confusion and outrage. We simply do not understand how the person can seem to be fine with everyone else but harsh or insensitive to us. Try to remember that this may happen because each of us has different memory networks dealing with work, friends and family. Different unprocessed memories can get triggered depending upon the type of relationship and the situation. If you and your partner are having problems, prepare yourself with a Safe/Calm Place and then try to identify together the situations and triggers. Commit to working on them together because both of you are necessary to make the relationship work. Consider using the Floatback technique to identify any memories that are running your show.

Practice generosity. Being generous with our partner means taking notice and offering time, assistance, a kind word or forgiveness for a minor slight. It involves reaching inside of ourselves to offer the best of what we have to the people we love. But to offer this, we also need to take care of ourselves. Make sure to use the self-help techniques you've already learned on a daily basis in order to nurture yourself and relieve stress.

Try to stay open. Sometimes when there has been a pattern of conflict, one can start to "shut down" and "close off" from a partner. It's almost like placing yourself in a steel box of sorts to prevent further damage. It's natural to want to protect yourself when you are hurt. But the problem with these boxes is that, while they may keep you "safe," they also isolate you and wall off any possibility for change. Sometimes it's a way to punish a partner, but it's also self-punishing, as you can feel numb, withdrawn and depressed. Notice how you feel in order to try to avoid closing down. Remember that you have choices. For instance, using the techniques you've learned can often help you to move from "closed" to "open"—relaxed, peaceful and interested.

Communicate. When it's time to talk with your partner about your patterns and how to change, make sure you are in an open state. Use statements such as "I love you, and when X happens, I feel Y." Not "You make me feel . . . !" We're all responsible for our own reactions. Share the information as you would like it shared with you. No blame, just information that is important to think and feel through together. If that doesn't work, remember to reach out for professional assistance to help evaluate the situation and offer useful choices. Sometimes it's important to have a specially trained neutral third party take a look with fresh eyes.

PERSONAL EXPLORATION

Jot down the three most disturbing personal or romantic relationship memories you have had since mid-adolescence. Which belief category do they fall into? Are they the same as or different than any of the belief statements you already identified? Use a Floatback to identify the child-hood memories that may be feeding your difficulties. Add them to your *Touchstone List.*

Consider whether any problems you're currently having in relationships can be dealt with through the communication skills and self-control techniques. If not, remember that if the current difficulties are the most recent example of others you've had in your life, seeking professional assistance to process the memories pushing your reactions may be a good option. Remember that you have choices.

A PART OF THE WHOLE

I mentioned in the first chapter that one purpose of this book was to better understand ourselves and those around us. I also said that it wasn't about assigning blame. But frankly, sometimes it's very hard not to do just that. Sometimes our sense of justice screams out, "THIS IS JUST WRONG!" We blame people who never seem to understand—especially when they hurt others over and over again. Sometimes people know that their actions are "wrong" by society's standards—but they do them anyway, without compassion or empathy. Others know their behavior is wrong and it bothers and shames them to do it, but they claim that they can't help themselves. Others think their actions are justified.

Not a day goes by when the newspapers aren't filled with tragedy that could have been prevented. We read about lives destroyed by people who seem to have no sense of responsibility for their actions. They just seem to walk through life smashing things—and people—around them. Nevertheless, the truth of the matter is that even here, judgment needs to be tempered with understanding. Because without understanding the why of it, we can't help bring about change. Yes, they should control themselves. Yes, they are often doing terrible harm. And yes, in most cases they can learn to do something about it. So we blame them even more: If they can learn to stop, then they should—but they don't!

We need to remember that *why* they aren't learning to control their destructive behavior is part of the problem that keeps them stuck. Unfortunately, as a society we have often given up on these people—and they've also given up on themselves. We may consider them either permanently damaged or unwilling to change. But neither of these views gets to the root of the problem or the possible solutions. The reasons for their actions are the same as everyone else's—automatic knee-jerk responses caused by unconscious processes. This doesn't excuse their actions. However, those who cause suffering are also part of the whole fabric of humanity. We may not like their destructive patterns. But, if we don't learn to understand and treat perpetrators successfully, we will continue to have victims. That's why in this chapter we'll look at child molesters, perpetrators of domestic violence, rapists and drug addicts. They may have already affected some of you directly or through a loved one. Ultimately, as a society, what they do affects us all—if for no other reason than we might be some of the people they end up hurting.

HOW DOES IT BEGIN?

There are many reasons for people to grow up to be what is called "antisocial."

Some say they can see the signs of it in "bad seeds"—children who act out in school and seem to be unreachable. But are they really?

One of these "bad seeds" turned up shortly after 9/11 when Gary arrived to start his job as an agency counselor at a rural elementary school. In tow was a brand-new play therapy bag full of well-used toys and art supplies—"expressive materials" as they are called—used to help children communicate their problems and feelings. In schools you tend to work where you can find space for it. His "office" was a big closet where the school stored textbooks and a media cart left over from the days when projectors were high-tech. So Gary cleared the cart and set up his toys and other supplies there. He didn't know EMDR therapy then, but he knew some play therapy techniques that had worked pretty well for him over the years.

One of Gary's first encounters that day was with Zach, a six-year-old boy who was repeating kindergarten. He and his brother and sister were living with a grandmother who was supporting them. Both parents had been caught dealing methamphetamine and were in prison. That seemed like significant information, but it didn't seem quite enough to explain Zach's behavior at school. The reason he was repeating kindergarten, and not too successfully, was that he was physically assaulting kids on the playground almost every day. This type of behavior, often diagnosed as a "conduct disorder," can lead to antisocial, violent behavior as an adult. Throughout the country these kinds of children are very often left back in school repeatedly, or pushed along even though they aren't learning. Many times they are incorrectly medicated or overmedicated to bring them into compliance. They often eventually drop out of school. With no skills and lots of anger, their lives generally go in predictable patterns.

At the end of their first play therapy session, Zach became enraged and threw all the toys off the cart and around the room. Gary said, "There must be some good reason you're having these strong feelings." Zach just ignored him. In fact, they did a couple of sessions like this where the child grabbed the neatly ordered play materials and flung them around the room.

Eventually Zach seemed to settle down and built a relationship with Gary. They worked together using play therapy. Yet after 20 sessions,

Zach was still acting out at school. Gary would often encounter him headed to the principal's office for more corporal punishment: head down, looking really tiny, getting ready to have a frustrated grown man swat him with a paddle. Corporal punishment was still a common practice in that part of the US. Although Gary talked with the principal, he couldn't stop him from doing what he thought he needed to do. Although he explained to the principal that there was a likely reason for Zach's puzzling behavior, it didn't help. Although Gary was doing his best, he couldn't get the reason out of the child.

A few months later, Gary traveled out of state for EMDR training. While there, he was able to talk to folks who worked with children. They told him the good thing about kids is that the treatment can often go very quickly. When he met with Zach two weeks later, he was able to show him how to use the Safe Place technique. And during the next session, everything changed. Five minutes before the end of the session, Zach began ripping all the toys off the media cart and heaving them around the room. He cleared the cart in about 60 seconds. Squatting on the floor facing each other, in the midst of scattered toys, Gary said, "Notice what you are feeling and where you feel it in your body," and using hand taps, he began EMDR processing.

Almost immediately Zach began crying from the gut, sobbing from his core. To Gary's amazement, Zach was more connected with his emotions in the four or five minutes on the floor than he had been in all their previous therapy. They did another round of processing that produced more sobbing and crying. Then Zach said, "It felt terrible when I was throwing the toys." Then he asked, "Can you keep a secret?"

Gary said, "Yes." He didn't know what he was going to hear. He braced himself for anything. Zach said among sobs, "My parents are in prison and they're not going to get out until I'm really old."

As they continued processing, Zach connected to his emotions and was able to feel them and express them. Then he focused on the memories of his parents that were feeding his strong feelings. During the processing Gary could see him making the emotional connections and having insights that he now could readily describe in words. This was a big shift in the underlying cause of the problem.

For many youngsters, some emotions are too much to bear. The brain's information processing system becomes overloaded, and the strong feelings are stored in a disconnected part of the memory. But something happening in the present can still trigger the emotions. For instance, at the end of each therapy session, Gary, the person Zach was now connected with, would be leaving him like his parents had. The feelings of pain, fear and anger fuel actions that seem out of control—throwing toys around the room or hurting other children as he did in the playground. Then the feelings subside and the child can't feel or express them. Children grow into adults that way, with the pain, anger and fear locked away but ready to explode.

The following week Gary spoke to Zach's teacher and found that he hadn't been in trouble and was doing well in class. He'd been having problems so long that it took his teacher and the other adults quite some time to accept that he was, in fact, getting better. Gary continued working with him using EMDR. One day he found out that Zach's grandmother had given his older brother back to the state permanently, because she didn't want him to be a bad influence on his siblings. He thought, "I'm going to have to start all over again." But he didn't. As they worked together that afternoon, Zach said, "My brother made bad choices. He's gone to a place where he can get help."

At the end of the school year, Zach graduated into first grade, and Gary was transferred to another district. He checked back with a colleague about Zach and heard that he was doing wonderfully. We don't know what happened to his brother. Let's hope he ran into a counselor like Gary who helped him through his pain.

The bottom line here is that many actions that hurt others, whether caused by children or adults, are based on earlier unprocessed memories that are running the show. Corporal punishment didn't change Zach's behavior. It just fueled the anger, pain and fear that were stored in his memory networks. His failure to graduate from kindergarten and all the schoolyard teasing that went along with it only added to the pain that caused him to act out in the first place. This is not to say that rules and discipline aren't important. Society has to set and enforce certain guidelines for everyone's safety. But the failure of parents to set the stage for healthy emotional development leaves many people with the inability to feel their emotions—or to self-soothe when they do. That leads to a whole range of problems, which we'll explore in this chapter.

IT'S GOT A HOLD ON ME

Because of their drug use, Zach's parents were not able to teach and guide him well. Addiction is not only a destructive problem on its own, it also often contributes to other negative behaviors we'll be looking at throughout this chapter. Drug and alcohol abuse is now viewed as a huge global health problem. And it's now commonly accepted that having an untreated trauma history can set the groundwork for the risk of substance abuse. Although there may be a genetic predisposition to addiction for some people, it generally takes certain kinds of life events to set the pattern of substance abuse in motion. The predisposition may make recovery more difficult—but genetics aren't destiny.

While some people are not in touch with their emotions, others are simply overwhelmed by them. When the pain becomes too much to bear, they turn outward for relief. Maybe they saw their parents cope that way, or maybe they just discovered they felt better after experimenting with drugs or alcohol with their peers. Whatever the reason, people who are addicted often feel out of control and powerless to stop regardless of how much they may want to or how many people they hurt. Thousands get behind the wheel when they're over the alcohol limit—with no intention other than to get from one place to another—and people are killed or permanently injured as a result. Whether the cause is an addiction or a one-time lapse of judgment, they shouldn't get behind the wheel in that state. But they do, and often someone suffers. Unfortunately, it's only after hitting rock bottom that many finally admit they need help.

It's Never Too Late

Substance addiction is a vicious circle. It can start out as a symptom of internal despair or worthlessness—but once it takes over, it only creates more cause for self-hatred as it takes its destructive course. To deal with addiction, it's important to learn different ways to manage emotional pain. But it's also important to process the earlier memories that are feeding the disturbance to begin with. A research study conducted in a Washington Drug Court Program combined EMDR therapy with a preparatory group treatment called Seeking Safety, which included education and skills for coping with trauma and substance abuse as well as self-soothing techniques. Preliminary data showed a 91.3% graduation rate from Drug Court for those voluntarily accepting EMDR treatment, compared to 62% for those who were eligible but declined it. More research is needed, but the results for the people in this integrated treatment program are clear. Graduating from Drug

Court is the best indicator of stopping the revolving door of drug use and jail time. The results show that regardless of how long or rough the addiction history, people can change for the better.

Tom has become an advocate for the EMDR Trauma Treatment program based on his experience in Drug Court. He has offered a description of his long journey "to hell and back" in the hope that it would help others in similar situations:

I started drinking at the age of 12, smoking pot at the age of 14 and then moving to harder drugs as time went by. Drinking and drugs made sense to me since I'd been watching my two alcoholic parents regularly drink their problems away. They were "great" parents; they were just alcoholics. And of course, my friends drank and used drugs, as did their parents.

I've been battling alcohol and drug addiction for 28 years. I've been to drug treatment four times, including 70 days incarcerated in a chemical dependency jail program that was part of my first attempt at Drug Court. That attempt was unsuccessful and resulted in three felony convictions, more jail time and the label of being a convicted felon. I hated that.

Tom had a good life mapped out for himself in his family's automotive and towing business, and loving parents who supported him in his life goals. But at 35, he watched his father battle cancer over a 2-year period, and that sent him into escalating drug and alcohol use. Then his father died.

Over the next year, I struggled with life, not knowing what to do. But then things started to look up when I landed a job for a large trucking company. Along with my brother Steve, who was my co-driver, we set out on a new career as long haul truck drivers. Everything seemed to be going OK, and for one year we successfully completed our assignments, driving through every state in the country. Then it happened, picking up a load in Texas on our way home for Christmas.

Steve and I stopped in the little town of Hays, Kansas, to do some Christmas shopping for our families. Afterwards, we went to the local bar for some "Christmas cheer." After closing down the bar and heading back to our truck, we began to fight about getting back on the road right away or waiting until morning. Steve wanted to go; I wanted to stay. I finally gave in and agreed to go, but as I eased our 80,000-pound truck out of the parking lot, our fight began to get very intense, yelling and screaming at the top of our lungs. I rolled onto the freeway on-ramp and started to pick up speed, the whole time yelling at my brother to shut up! We went on and on, screaming and cursing at each other, neither of us able to just stop the fight. That's when he screamed at the top of his lungs, "Maybe I should just get out right here!" And at the top of my lungs I yelled the last words I ever spoke to my brother: "Go ahead!" I slipped the truck into high gear at 65 mph; my brother calmly sat back, undid his seat belt, unlocked his door and stepped out of the truck. It took almost a quarter-mile to stop that 18-wheeler. I ran down the road, finally coming upon my brother facedown in a ditch, bones sticking out everywhere and a river of blood flowing out of his broken body. He died in my arms.

Of course, I dealt with the tragic death of my brother the only way I knew how—with drugs and alcohol. I was in trouble, and I knew it. With the love and support of my mother, I entered into my first inpatient treatment program. Unfortunately, after a few short months of recovery, I went right back to what seemed to work best—substances, though never enough to touch the pain they were intended to extinguish.

Over the next few years Tom couldn't keep a job, was divorced, lost his mother to alcohol-induced liver failure, and ran through all his money on drugs. Then he was arrested for methamphetamine possession and driving on a suspended license.

Over the next year I would be arrested and booked 13 more times. I would get arrested, bailed out, miss my court dates, and go on "warrant status," hiding out and running from the cops. They would come to my house, kick my front door in, hold my family at gunpoint, and search my house looking for me. My biggest fear was not going to jail. It was knowing that as soon as I got arrested, I wouldn't be able to do dope. I was terminated from the Drug Court program, sentenced on three felonies, and did my time.

After his release, Tom went right back to using drugs and was arrested and jailed again. This time while on probation and facing another jail term if he used, he accepted the chance to enter the Drug Court's EMDR Trauma Treatment research program. Over the next five months he worked on the "core issues" of his addiction, and he wants people to know that it made his recovery possible.

Because he wants others to try EMDR treatment, he's offering a look at his life now:

In the six years of my recovery, I've completely turned my life around. I paid off over $10,000 in court fines, got my driver's license reinstated, pulled my house out of foreclosure, paid off my attorney, completed all my probation. I have successfully owned and operated my own business for one and a half years and I pay all my bills. I am now a responsible and accountable member of society, and the best part is, I have a family that includes my fiancée, who now has 19 months of recovery, my 17-year-old daughter, who has moved back home with us, and my 8-year-old daughter, who always makes my life interesting. I now look forward to each and every day.

Many people believe that addiction is simply a lack of "discipline." They don't understand how a person's life can just spiral out of control to this degree. I hope Tom's story helps clarify that. When people use alcohol or drugs to handle their emotions, the substances can take on a life of their own. But once the unprocessed memories that are pushing the addiction are handled, life can turn around again. Don't let shame about your past lock you in place and ruin your future. Seek out the help you need to make responsible new choices. Even after almost three decades of battling his demons, Tom's story shows that it's never too late to make the choices and changes needed to lead a healthy life.

Searching for the Source

The EMDR treatment that Tom received included processing (1) the past memories feeding his disturbance, (2) the current situations that triggered the desire to use drugs, and (3) new ways to deal with disturbing experiences. To prevent relapse, it's important to process the earlier memories that are pushing the pain. In Tom's case they included major traumas, such as the death of his brother and his overwhelming sense of responsibility for causing his death. For others with addictions, even with major events in their lives, the most important memory can be something unsuspected.

For instance, Karen had been suffering from panic attacks for as long as she could remember. She dealt with them by multiple drug use and sexual addiction. Ten years of therapy hadn't stopped the panic attacks, and as much as she tried, she couldn't kick her addictions either. Finally arriving at an EMDR clinician, they targeted the feelings of fear in her body, and her mind went back to something that happened when she was four years old. Her parents dropped her off at the park with her two-year-old sister and told Karen to take care of her. It seemed like forever before they returned, and by the time they did Karen was in a full-blown panic, vomiting and sobbing in fear. Instead of comforting her, her father just yelled at her—and then laughed at her for acting like a "wimp." The fear, shame and lack of control encoded in this memory set the stage for her addictions. She took her first sip of beer at the age of five and went on from there. As is often the case, Karen's parents were "misattuned" to her needs and gave her no support, sense of confidence or positive, constructive ways to manage distress. Tom, on the other hand, described "loving" and "great" parents who supported him. But they taught him to drink by "modeling" that the way to deal with negative emotions and problems was to "drink them away." In either case, whatever the cause of the addiction, the road to recovery is clear: It involves dealing with pain straight on—finding new ways to view the past, deal with the present and make plans for the future. Without addressing these powerful seeds of addiction, things will likely only get worse.

When There's Nowhere Else to Go

One of the clinicians who now works for the EMDR-Humanitarian Assistance Programs once ran a homeless outreach center. They offered addiction treatment on demand to the people who wanted it, as well as other types of assistance—winter coats, referrals for medical care, or food. At some point, all her clients would ask if life would get better after they got sober. She told them that it would, as it was the truth. She knew that they would gain access to safer housing, increase their chances of finding and keeping a job, and perhaps have the opportunity to reconnect with the people they loved. But she knew that without the blanket of soothing chemicals to cover their pain, it was also going to be hard—very hard—as all of them had endured years of trauma. In particular, she worried about the men and women whose addictions had cost them their children, as well as the people who had been sexually and physically abused both on the street and in their own homes as youngsters.

Years have passed since then, and now there is a greater understanding of addiction as a disease and how past trauma feeds the destructive processes. She now uses EMDR therapy in a private practice and continues to see people with severe substance abuse problems. As she tells it:

Yesterday, one of my clients, who had been doing better, came in slightly intoxicated and upset due to a recent loss. At one point, she looked in my eyes and asked me straight out—"Will I feel lovable one day? Will I ever be able to accept a partner who will love and care for me?"

I thought of the work she had already accomplished using EMDR—leaving an abusive alcoholic husband, lengthy periods of abstinence from alcohol use herself, surviving and coping with rape, sexual abuse and neglect that started at age five and persisted throughout her adulthood—and I said, with assurance, "Yes, you are going to get there." Gone was any of the internal hesitation I used to feel in my homeless outreach days. I knew she would definitely reach her desired destination, but in fact she couldn't yet see what I could— that she had already made half the journey. For when she called for a ride home from therapy, a reliable, caring friend—someone who loves her—eagerly offered to bring her home. Despite the odds, her life was getting better, and I knew I could help her." Yes, help is available. But to get it, you need enough of a glimmer of hope to show up.

Learning to Connect

Not all people turn to drugs to deal with their negative emotions. Some deal with it through excessive use of pornography, sex, gambling, food or any number of different experiences that allow a temporary feeling of distraction, calm or satisfaction. But there are so many other healthy ways to achieve long-lasting positive feelings. Addictive behaviors are just temporary fixes that don't last because they don't get to the root of the problem. Once the "high" is gone, the negative feelings come back.

For anyone who has grown up in a family feeling lonely, isolated, not good enough—or who never learned how to deal with strong negative emotions—the risks are clear. Dealing effectively with addictions means not only addressing the sources of the pain, but also learning the tools to deal with disturbing emotions when they arise and learning new ways to interact with people.

People who have been traumatized as children are significantly more likely than the rest of the population to develop an addiction. Because of their pain and the feeling that they're "different," they don't fit in with their peers and don't learn the social skills necessary for healthy relationships. Without therapy, they often cannot make the connections necessary for recovery. For instance, the sense of community, feeling welcomed, and the openness and honesty in a 12-Step Program can be very useful. But some people also need EMDR therapy to help them deal with the program's requirements, because being with groups of people or being expected to "disclose" things about themselves triggers feelings of shame and insecurity. As you may suspect by now, these feelings are rooted in earlier life experiences that need to be processed. The bottom line is that no matter how many times someone may have failed before, it's worth trying again with the right help. As you can see from Tom's experience, there is a way.

PUTTING ON A MASK

One of the first men I ever worked with came in for therapy because of difficulties he had in social situations. As Jose described it, when he was around people he had *"a fear that comes over me that is so intense it interrupts whatever is going on at the moment, and it just overpowers me to a point where I want to run and hide."* When I asked him to put the feelings into words, he said, *"I just feel different—like I don't belong."* He said he wanted help because *"It seems like it's taken such a major part of my life that it's caused me to get into the ways of alcohol and drugs to get rid of it. I just numb myself to the point where I don't feel that experience anymore. But that pain is coming up especially hard now that I'm trying to recover from the addictions."*

Jose grew up thinking, *"What's wrong with me?"* As he described it, *"I have a younger brother. When we were growing up he was the favorite. He was always better at everything and he was accepted more. He had everything more. My stepfather at the time—my real father I didn't know—liked him more. He gave him credit for everything more and it affected me so much to where I was crying for attention. I guess I was trying to do everything I could, and I would fumble things up sort of in an awkward way to try to get some sort of attention. To say to my stepfather, 'Hey, look. I'm here too. You know. I do a lot of good things also. Some even better.' I hated my brother. He had more girlfriends and I mean it got to the point where it affected me so much that I got so shy and felt, heck, who wanted to talk to me? So as a result, I gave him a lot of power, I guess."*

When I asked Jose where else the fear came up, he said, *"Gang fights. Juvenile hall. Jail. Fights with my brothers."* With more questioning, he explained: *"The fear that I had—the feeling that I had about myself—being different. Not liked. Not getting attention. I guess it made me think that I was different and that I didn't belong there and I questioned myself. So that would just lead to misunderstandings. The hatred that developed would always cause a misunderstanding between my brothers and my sisters and me. So as a result, we would just have a knock-down-drag-out."*

When I asked about juvenile hall, he explained, *"Juvenile hall would come up—this goes back when I was growing up in Texas as a teenager. It still goes on now but in Texas there was a big heavy metal thing with North against South—turfs they called them. Me and my other brother sort of got involved in that growing up and there was always one turf against another turf, or one turf being on another's turf and getting ran out in one form or another. And that is when the juvenile hall would come in."*

I asked him, "How would the feeling of the fear of being different get you involved?" Jose explained, *"I found the gang to be something that I could get accepted in, that I was accepted in. And that is where the alcohol came into the scene. It gave me false courage to deal with those feelings. I strangely bought into that. Being macho. Tramping around. Drinking. Saying cuss words. Smoking. Making fun of people and hurting people. I felt accepted there. I mean, that is the only way I could deal with life then. Sort of like a survival. Otherwise the thought of doing myself in would occur every now and then."*

Jose is pretty typical of those who resort to violence because of underlying feelings of anger and pain. While many people believe that those who seem to feel no empathy and have no hesitation in hurting others are "psychopaths" who cannot be treated, recent research has indicated that is not always the case. Our overcrowded prisons are loaded with people who have had childhoods that left them feeling isolated. Since we all need some sense of identification, gangs often substitute as "family." Whether in a gang or not, the absence of support by their parents—being pushed away, abandoned, humiliated or beaten—that results in feeling not good enough leaves them ripe to hurt other people. Jose was doing the same thing Zach did.

If you feel abandoned, worthless or different in your own family, how do you identify with the rest of society? And if you don't identify with society, why obey the rules? Make up your own—that way you're in charge and you get to do the hurting. It can end up in very scary places. But the start is generally the same—a vulnerable, angry and confused child. Processing their memories liberated Zach and Jose from their pain and feelings of isolation. It's better to do it early, at Zach's age—for both the child and society. But as seen with Jose and Tom, even a prison record doesn't mean it's too late.

HOUSE OF PAIN

Just as it's easy to look at gang members on the street and buy into the image of "Don't mess with me" power and control they are trying to project, the same is true of perpetrators of domestic violence. As we've already seen, some couples participate equally in a destructive dance of jealousy, criticism, manipulation and frustration. However, physical domestic violence in a relationship is generally a one-way street. Although some women are also offenders, by and large about 85% of those who use violence are men. It's also not as rare as you might think. In fact, one of the most quoted reasons for women becoming homeless is domestic violence.

In general, an abusive man's behavior can involve an ongoing intention to scare, hurt or destroy his partner or anything that belongs to her. This is not a one-time overload fueled by drugs or alcohol. There's often a sense of "entitlement." The abusive partner exerts power to control the woman's behavior to ensure her compliance. She's there to please and comfort him. Violence often occurs in a three-stage process. Tension builds, the man explodes in rage, and finally he expresses his love and tries to make it up to her in a "honeymoon" period. This cycle repeats again and again. It's been reported that domestic violence is one of the leading causes of injury and death worldwide in women ages 19–44.

Generally, it's the woman who comes in for help because life has become unmanageable. Most often she describes feelings of depression, anxiety or concern for the children. In Marie's case, the breaking point came when Jacques became physically violent with their eight-year-old son at his birthday party and used a knife to scare them both. He had never done that. Before, he had been violent only with her and without a weapon. She finally decided to leave. It was a difficult decision for her, and she knew the danger of him becoming increasingly violent, so she left while he was at work. As Jacques later told his clinician, when he found out she was gone, "I looked for her everywhere." In response to the question "Why?" he replied, "To kill her and to shoot myself afterwards. But then I thought about my children, and I didn't do it. I started to calm down after three days."

Basically, Jacques felt that he couldn't live without Marie. Because of that, he would experience a high level of fear whenever she tried to express some independence. For instance, he used to take all the phones in the house to work with him because he couldn't understand why she needed to talk to anyone other than him. According to Jacques, "If she loves me as I love her, she doesn't need to talk with anybody else. If she does it, that's because she wants to hide something from me." These types of actions are typical of domestic abusers. They try to isolate their partners by controlling their resources, access to friends, or other aspects of daily life.

Marie accepted Jacques' behavior because she had very low self-esteem. She also came from a family in which women were trained to take care of men. Her job was to feed him, dress him—she chose the clothes he wore every day—and be available to him. Just as she tried to earn her parents' love by "doing" for them, she told her therapist that she couldn't have been involved in a relationship with someone who didn't need her to take care of him. Both of them were repeating behavior patterns learned within their families of origin: Men didn't do anything at home; women did everything. Men didn't exist by themselves, and women thought that their lives were meant to take care of their husbands.

Not really in touch with their feelings or with the skills to express them, Jacques would often explode, Marie would cower, and often she would get hurt. In many ways, feeling as though she was "walking on eggshells," Marie was hypervigilant—in a constant state of fear and high alert. She had what some clinicians have described as "brain freeze." Her logical, rational mind wasn't really online. It was similar to the way animals in the wild "freeze" or "flee" when confronted by danger. And when escape is impossible, they collapse. So when Jacques became violent, Marie just took it.

She was also in a state that other clinicians refer to as "learned helplessness." Nothing she could do would make a difference. After all, she had learned that men were supposed to get their way with women. She loved Jacques and believed she couldn't live without him. She believed he would never really hurt her "too much." As with many other victims of domestic violence, Marie wasn't able to act until something broke the pattern. It wasn't until Jacques became violent with their son and grabbed the knife that Marie could no longer tolerate his actions and left.

After leaving the house, she lived in a women's shelter with their two children. She and Jacques had been separated for six months when she heard a clinician speak about domestic violence on the radio. She called to make an appointment for Jacques with the description "He's a little nervous and has a short temper." He hadn't yet taken responsibility for his violent behavior and most likely would come to see a therapist just to please her. The therapist told her that Jacques would need to call and make his own appointment.

When Jacques came in to meet the therapist, he said that he wanted to try to understand what happened to him and what he could do to get his wife back. Did he think he was violent? "Not really, just a very jealous man with a short fuse. I did everything for her. I built our house; I gave her my money." He clearly didn't understand what was happening within himself—but he agreed that he was hurting Marie. How long had the violence gone on? "Nineteen years," he replied. Then Jacques confessed that he respected Marie more now that she had left: "She showed me she could do it. Before, she always talked about it but never did it. I'm proud of her." Although when she left, Jacques originally tried to find Marie with the intention of killing both of them, his reaction at this point wasn't unusual. Now she was no longer there to care for him and make him feel safe. When she left, he felt completely powerless and out of control, and he needed to find a solution within himself.

With both now living in separate apartments, the therapy lasted a year. It included EMDR, plus couples and family therapy and group sessions. There were multiple goals, which included developing a greater level of self-esteem and healthy attachment for both of them, as well as learning the communication skills necessary in an adult relationship. In addition, Jacques needed to process his early memories of violence in his original family and increase his ability to deal with strong emotion. Marie needed to learn how to exist contentedly without him and to take care of herself. She realized that in her original family, she "always came way after everyone else."

A few of the targets they each processed with EMDR therapy are very revealing of the unconscious memory processes that were running their show. The first major target for Jacques was his last violent outburst when he threatened his son with a knife. The major insight he gained from this was that he had never known how to be a father. The only person who counted for him was his wife. The children were always in the middle. Then he targeted another very important memory of himself as an eight-year-old child. He was with his family and he wanted to help his mom by bringing the food to the dinner table. His father, in a very violent way, yelled at him, "Sit down, only gay guys get up to help." He remembered being frozen by the remark and not knowing what to do.

Other important memories for Jacques involved being afraid that his mother didn't love him, and always trying to attract her attention. He realized, "If I had felt more safely loved by her, I wouldn't have to be so dependent on my wife's love." Therapy also included targeting ways in which he could live alone, nurture himself and be less dependent on his wife—including going to see a movie on his own, while his wife spent time with some friends.

For Marie, the initial target was the first time Jacques had been violent with her. She had been pregnant with their first child and remembered how "He hit me on my tummy, knowing the baby was inside." The major insight for her was realizing that he was "sick with too much inappropriate jealousy" and that she couldn't do anything about it. She had to learn to protect herself. Another key target was: "He always asked me to go in front of the light when we were going out to check if he could see through my dress." Since she always carefully checked herself, she realized then how she let him control her. She went on to process the control issues she had seen between her parents. Her dad controlling her mom with money, the car, TV programs—and her mom controlling her dad with how to dress, the food to eat, the children and all the emotional decisions. She realized on a gut level that she had to let go of the need to control and be controlled. She needed to discover and experience freedom for herself.

Of course their children had not been spared the effects of the violence. EMDR therapy was needed to help their daughter, who started to show delinquent behavior at school. Their son had started behaving like Dad with his sister, using physical violence. Family therapy sessions helped stop this acting out and set up new communication patterns. Both parents had to change their parenting styles, and Marie had to learn to intervene with the children and not to wait for Jacques' reaction.

To understand domestic violence, it's important to remember that it's a complex situation that can involve family history, unresolved trauma or other cultural factors. Often the feelings of powerlessness and helplessness stem from early trauma histories. At the beginning of treatment, both Marie and Jacques shared the same negative cognitions: "I am worthless" and "I am stupid." Both were afraid to exist without the other. Both shared the same level of insecure attachment because of psychological and physical (for him) violence in their families of origin. At the end of treatment, both described a general feeling of freedom, as if something had been lifted to allow them all to live and breathe. They moved back in together, and they have lived together in peace for many years.

Other couples may not be able to maintain the effort and commitment needed to heal. For a family to emerge intact, it's critical that the batterer participate fully in treatment. It's useful for all members to see if therapy is necessary. Often the victim needs to process memories of the abuse. It's also vital that the children be evaluated carefully because they often take on the blame for their parents' flaws. Without therapy, they may slip into the same patterns as their parents, as they may carry the feelings of guilt and insecurity within them.

For instance, here's a statement from a young girl who used to hide under the covers with her brother, listening to their mother sob and scream as her husband beat her. Bonnie started EMDR therapy saying,

It feels like the world is closing in on me, and a black hole has swallowed me up. Because of Dad, everything has gone black. In processing the worst memory, which she said made her feel as though her "heart was ripped apart," each set of eye movements brought her new understanding:

>> *I felt really guilty and thought it was my fault being really naughty and getting him angry and that's why it happened.*

>>*I just thought I did something really bad without really noticing it and got my dad really angry. But come to think of it, I don't think it's my fault. If I'd done anything wrong, he would come to hit me and not Mum.*

>> *I don't think Mum did anything wrong. I think Dad might just have been drinking.*

After more processing, Bonnie is now liberated from her pain, but she doesn't forgive her father for what he did. Whether or not the family is reunited will depend on many factors. One of the most important is a clear change in her father's attitude and behaviors.

SEXUAL ABUSERS

There is nothing that turns people's stomachs more than the thought of child sexual abuse. Again, while some women are perpetrators, most are men—and too many children are affected. There are daily stories in the newspapers of children being molested by teachers, coaches and youth leaders of various sorts. In fact, research has reported that approximately 20% of girls and 10% of boys worldwide have been molested. It's also disturbing that evaluations of the most widespread treatments for abusers have shown disappointing results. That's why many states demand that child molesters be tracked for life, often with satellite bracelets to monitor their whereabouts. There's the feeling that these people are just too sick to be cured. One of the problems is the programs that are most generally used have not changed very much over the past 20 years. They primarily involve group therapy to help clarify motives, learning skills to self-monitor in order to avoid situations where deviant sexual feelings might be triggered, and then techniques to try to get rid of the desire. One of the reasons these programs often don't work may be because the treatment deals with only the behavior, as opposed to also dealing with the cause of the behavior.

While group therapy and self-monitoring can be useful, the problem is that the abuser is often not really able to participate. Group therapy is supposed to help the abuser take responsibility for what he did and clarify his motives. But one of the symptoms of abusers is "denial"—they often simply believe that their actions weren't really their fault, and they didn't actually hurt anyone. Despite the best efforts of treatment providers to break through denial, offenders often learn to say the right things even though they may continue to maintain deeply held mistaken beliefs. This can come about because they are not in touch with their feelings due to their own abuse histories. It turns out that many people who are child molesters were victims of child abuse themselves. That in no way means that everyone who has been molested will molest other people. Far from it. But it means that when certain conditions come into play, a history of having been abused appears to be a contributing factor.

As you've already seen in this book, a traumatic experience becomes locked into the brain with the emotions, thoughts and feelings that were there at the time of the event. When children are abused, there are a number of faulty perceptions they can carry away from the experience. For example, the child may feel: *This is the way life is. This is what I have to do in order to get love and attention. This is a good way to get what I want. I hated it but it made me stronger,* and so forth. Basically, there is a wide range of reactions that may contribute to the emotions and unspoken beliefs that can later drive the sexual offending.

Unfortunately, many children who have been molested blame themselves for the assault, just as Bonnie blamed herself while her father was beating her mother. In addition, unlike a rape that is generally a sudden show of force, anger and power, molesters often "groom" their victims. While some terrorize youngsters into complying with threats, others take another approach. They do things to make their chosen victims feel good before the molestation begins. When children come from a family in which they are made to feel unimportant or unwanted, receiving so much attention is a new and pleasurable experience for them. As a result, they may go along with whatever the molester wants. Then, since healthy bodies often react to physical stimulation, if theirs do, molesters tell their victims they really like what happened and that they actually caused it—and the children believe them. This also confuses the child's sense of trust and feelings about what is right and wrong in adult-child relationships.

Many times, with the shame and guilt then locked into the memory stored in their brain, molested children can "remember" that they "wanted it" and it's their fault. So, instead of anger and blame being directed at the perpetrator, the victim directs it inward. "It's my fault—I caused it!" Then if they molest others when they become an adult, it becomes a straight line to blaming their own victims. "It's his fault. He really wanted it." "I did it because she was a little flirt. She enjoyed it." For many people, the physical sensations that were locked into the brain also become triggered when they see a child. The new victim is often the same age as they were at the time of the original assault. Add to that the fact that many of these molesters come from homes where they were ignored and abused. They never learned to deal with their emotions and often end up not even being in touch with their feelings. This is where EMDR treatment comes in.

A study of child molesters who were in a program that used a traditional approach that included group therapy and self-monitoring techniques was published in the *Journal of Forensic Psychiatry and Psychology*. Ten perpetrators who had been molested themselves as children were treated with an additional eight sessions of EMDR directed at the memory of their own abuse. The results were compared to other molesters who hadn't received EMDR therapy, and the benefits were clear in nine of the ten molesters. For the first time, men took full responsibility for what they'd done. Instead of blaming their victims, they realized the damage they had caused. And, most importantly, the researchers used a device called a "penile plethysmograph," which uses the blood flow to the penis in order to physically measure sexual arousal. Researchers and clinicians see that as the prime sign of whether someone will offend again. This test showed that in nine of ten offenders, their sexual arousal to children steeply declined. The offenders explained their decreased arousal by describing that they now viewed children as "people" rather than as "sexual objects." The results were the same when they were retested a year later. More research is planned, but since that time, many perpetrators have been successfully treated with EMDR therapy.

It's important to understand the causes of a problem if we're going to solve it. For the first time, the perpetrators who were treated with EMDR were able to get in touch with the feelings they had experienced when they were molested themselves. It changed them—and now they want to encourage others to also get treatment. We'll start with Kevin, who molested his stepdaughter. He had been sodomized by a group of older boys when he was a youngster. He had been convinced he'd caused it. During processing he was able to get in touch with his feelings about the event. He remembered seeing someone walk past the shed while the assault was happening, and he was able to feel the loneliness and pain he experienced at that time. He recognized that he liked the attention he had been getting from the older boys, and they'd used him. But also, for the first time, he realized that his stepdaughter had liked attention too— but not the sexual act.

Here's how he explains what changed for him because of the EMDR processing of his own molestation:

I was still blaming myself for what happened, as well as putting blame on my victim like she was the one who caused this now. Up until this, thinking of what happened to me, I thought, "You're not a victim, because you brought this on to yourself. You was asking for it." But I didn't do jack squat. I didn't do nothing. I didn't cause it. And it helped me to have insight into my own abuse and see that it wasn't my fault. No more than it was my victim's fault. It's hard. It's hard to look at. But, the more you do, the more clear you become on what you did, as well as reality. Once you do see it clear, you can go back and say, "Oh, why in the world did I do this?" Or "How in the world could they do this to me?" and "How could I do this to them?" And that hurts. It's a big reality check. I had no understanding of feelings, of my own feelings. To be able to understand theirs, I had to really be able to understand mine. And once I could understand mine, I could understand theirs.

Also being able to feel somebody else's hurt. It's like that movie we watched the other day, The Accused. *I got pissed, I got really pissed, because hell, they were making her out to be the perpetrator. I mean, hell, she was the victim. And they were making her the criminal. Before the treatment, I'd have said, "She went in that bar. She went in there looking like that. She got what she deserved. She shouldn't have gone in there to start with." But even if she was a prostitute and she had had sex with four people, if I came up and she said, "Nah, I don't want to"— raping her would be wrong, because she didn't want it. But I never looked at it like that before.*

Louis is another perpetrator who was imprisoned for molesting his stepdaughter and also confessed to a number of rapes. An uncle who was 20 years his senior began molesting him around age 10. Then, in turn, he started acting out with boys his own age that he knew from school. At the age of 17 Louis left home to enlist in the armed services and was sent overseas. While there, he began having frequent sex with prostitutes, women he would meet in bars, and men who would pay him. After he returned to the US, he committed four rapes. He'd meet women at parties, take them to a private place, and force them to have sex.

Louis later married and became a father to his wife's two young children. As his stepdaughter neared puberty, around the time he'd been molested, Louis began to engage her in horseplay. He became sexually aroused during those times—shifting between feeling shame at his reaction and anger at her for "putting out sexual energy." Eventually Louis began to sexually touch her. This behavior continued and escalated for a number of months. Meanwhile, he became more and more verbally aggressive with his wife and the children. His wife insisted they all go to counseling. In the course of that therapy, his stepdaughter disclosed the sexual abuse. Louis was arrested, charged and imprisoned. He completed a treatment program and was released into the community under court supervision. Although he started outpatient sex offender therapy and seemed "motivated," he made little progress. He still believed that the females "put out sexual energy," which caused him to offend. Then he entered the EMDR treatment program.

During EMDR processing, Louis got in touch with the rage and shame he had experienced at the time of his own molestation. Thinking that nobody cared about him, he didn't really care about anyone else. He also realized that his distorted belief about "putting out sexual energy" came from the idea that he'd somehow brought on his own abuse. Instead, it became clear to him that his uncle had manipulated and used him. In turn, this led him to a sense of responsibility as well as real remorse for what he had done to his stepdaughter. His group members noticed how differently he was responding—how much more empathy and concern he showed. But he still wasn't thinking clearly about the rapes he had committed.

Additional processing of targets got him in touch with his feelings of rage toward his mother. Not only had she turned a blind eye to his father's drunken physical abuse of him, she'd caused him extreme humiliation. He had been a frequent bed wetter into his early teens (while he was being molested) and this was a source of shame and conflict in the family. His mother would become enraged with him, rub the urine-soaked sheets in his face and on his body, and send him to school smelling of it in an effort to stop him. Once Louis was able to successfully process his rage toward his mother and females in general, he took full responsibility for the rapes as well. It's important here to recognize that Louis' actions as a molester and his actions as a rapist needed to be targeted separately, as they were linked to different sets of memories. This underscores the need to evaluate all the pathways to different kinds of sexual abuse. Although Louis' victims were primarily adults, he was initially most puzzled by the physical reactions he had as a child molester. Here's how Louis describes his therapy experience:

After I got out of prison, I wanted to understand why I had molested my stepdaughter and why as an adult I was attracted to a child. Why did I get an erection around a child?

What I realized is that I got stuck as a child emotionally in that process of being molested. And also I didn't have a love connection with my parents. There were eight children in the household. Everyone was stressed out with their part of what they had to do to keep the assembly line going. I didn't have a one-on-one relationship with my mom or dad. So I couldn't go to my parents and tell them I was being molested.

When I did the EMDR, I went from the child with those experiences over to the adult side. Then I realized how I was able to molest and date-rape with the anger, shame and guilt associated with that child. All of my adult life I was an immature adult with the emotions of a child letting those emotions serve me, and they didn't serve me well. I ended up hurting a lot of people, going to prison, destroying lives.

WHY IT MATTERS

The bottom line here is that unprocessed memories cause people to react to their world through the emotions, beliefs and physical sensations that were there at the time of their earlier traumatic experiences. Sometimes they are the only ones hurt—by feeling danger when it's not there and experiencing phobias, depression or panic attacks. At other times, people harm others. Some act out of pain, rage, hate or despair and don't care who gets hurt. Others don't even understand that what they are doing is wrong. That's not an excuse. But it is an explanation. As members of a society, we are all part of a whole. The "worst" among us can hurt the most vulnerable among us. We have much more research and investigation to do over the next decade in all of these areas. But so far, the evidence is pointing to the possibility of not having to give up on anyone. And that's good news for all of us.

I'm not saying that all people can be successfully treated at this time.

There's a lot more to learn. For instance, some research is indicating that traumatic brain injuries can also contribute to criminal behavior. But the destructive behavior of millions of people who commit crimes is driven by treatable mental health problems. The reasons may have come from childhood, or trauma can sneak up on them as an adult and shake their very core. Sam is a good example of that. He was an inmate who came to the prison psychologist because he was having panic attacks whenever there was a plane crash on TV. Sam had been a cop—a good one. According to him, he "worked for the people." It was his job "to keep them safe no matter what." Every day he'd go the extra mile, patrol on foot, come early and stay late. Then he saw a horrendous plane crash in his city that took out 12 square blocks.

As he told the prison therapist, he'd gone to a thousand tragic scenes such as accidents, and had seen many, many injuries and deaths. But this one got to him—so badly that he ended up quitting his job and, over a ten-year period, sank lower and lower until he finally began committing crimes that put him in the federal prison system. He said the "nuclear-looking landscape where there used to be neighborhoods" haunted him the most. Then there were the things that were together but "shouldn't have been": a chair, a table with a glass of water still on it, and a torso. A doll, an arm with a ring still on the hand, and a children's book. Things like that.

Their EMDR target was the "nuclear landscape." The first set of eye movements resulted in the picture spontaneously changing to where it was still dismal but "cleaned up," with the debris gone. The next set startled Sam, as he saw green grass and trees growing there. The therapist said, "Stay with that." During the next set, he saw that a park had been built. He'd forgotten that had happened. Then he could calmly remember the incident with the major focus being that he could not have done anything about it, and that the area was repaired and rebuilt for the joy of future residents.

Sam no longer had panic attacks when he saw plane crashes on TV. He also returned to his devoted, "decent" self. As with the others in this chapter, whether their crimes are large or small, it is important to remember that they are a part of our society. As stated in a recent review article published in the medical journal *Lancet*, "Mental illness, which increases the risk of crime and repeat offending, is common in prisoners." Treating the mental health problems driving so many of them protects and strengthens us all. By treating perpetrators, we help them connect with a shared sense of humanity. And we can help stop the creation of more victims.

Sam said that the memory of a good place arising from a totally destroyed one served as a worthwhile metaphor for his own life. And I think it serves as a good metaphor for us all. Whether the horrendous nuclear landscape comes as an adult or from childhood—it can be transformed. We just have to do our best to get the help we need to turn it around. And try to get it to those who don't know enough to ask.

CHAPTER

IO

FROM STRESSED TO BETTER THAN WELL

Whether we are dealing with our family, work or other facets of life—those things we haven't examined or processed may push us in directions that cause pain and unhappiness. Dealing with those things directly can liberate us to enjoy life. Some of us are dealing with long-standing problems, while others are facing new situations that are difficult to understand. Some of the problems are confined to one area of our lives, and others seem all-encompassing, poisoning every area of our existence. Either way, you can benefit by using the techniques you've learned in this book to develop an understanding of why you are feeling and responding to the world in certain ways—and what to do about it.

In this chapter, we'll continue our exploration of the hidden landscape of the unconscious, and learn additional ways to deal with stress in our lives. I'll also explain some techniques that performers, executives and athletes use to excel. Basically, life is not just about getting rid of suffering. It's about expanding our potential while embracing feelings of joy and well-being.

STRESSED TO THE MAX

We have no control over our genetics, our childhood or, often, the current situations that arise in our lives. However, even when there is a genetic predisposition, in most cases problems arise or intensify because of an interaction between this predisposition and current life experiences. Research has actually shown that stress can negatively affect our genes, even damaging them to the point of shortening our life span. It can also have a negative effect on the brain itself. Our best course is to find ways to reduce the stress in our lives. In many instances, the primary cause is the unprocessed memories that are running us. However, the good news is: It doesn't have to take years to identify and correct the problems. We can learn to take more control of our own bodies and minds. That can allow us to make a difference in how we see the world. It can also help change the reactions that may draw us to the types of situations that cause us stress or that make it worse.

So let's take a look at stress from two areas that we all deal with. The first example focuses on family, the second on the workplace. We'll then cover additional personal control techniques, including some that are recommended by athletic and executive coaches. The following stories are examples of how we create the world we live in.

Why Did You Leave Me?

In an earlier chapter I mentioned that research has indicated that many people suffering from panic disorders were separated from their parents for some period of time when they were youngsters. But symptoms are not always cut-and-dried. Many people who have panic attacks do not have that history. And many people who have been separated do not develop a panic disorder. Instead, they may have other symptoms that can poison their existence. Frank's life is an example of how these unprocessed memories of childhood can set the foundation for a wide range of problems. In Frank's case, this led to poor choices, unsuccessful relationships as an adult and an array of other symptoms. Notice how many symptoms Frank has and see if any relate to you.

At 55 years old, Frank needed to deal with the overwhelming stress he experienced in his life. He came into therapy complaining of frequent headaches, forgetfulness, angry outbursts, irritability, sadness and feelings of insecurity. He was quite overweight and also suffered from diabetes, high blood pressure and chronic back pain.

"I am a very controlling person," Frank admitted to his therapist. "I need to be in control at all times." He didn't trust other people very much, including his current wife, Arlene, and his children. He was afraid of failure, especially in his personal relationships. He also experienced a fear of intimacy and low self-esteem. Pushed by his inner world, Frank was a people-pleaser. He felt that if he kept everyone around him happy they wouldn't abandon him. In reality, they all did. His two ex-wives and his children all left in various ways. He had been married three times and desperately wanted his present marriage to work. He was afraid that Arlene would divorce him if she really got to know who he was, so he tried to keep most of his emotions and opinions to himself.

Unfortunately, when we try to stuff down our emotions they often come out sideways. He reported a repeating cycle of directing explosive anger toward Arlene, just as he'd done with his previous wives. A potential conflict would start, tension would build, usually he would be the one to "blow up," and then hurt feelings and more anger would appear. Frank and Arlene would then distance themselves from each other. Days later they would reconcile without resolving the original problem. Frank commented, "I'm not able to talk about the issues that arise between us. I just lash out in anger when the hurt becomes too much to bear. All I can think about is protecting myself."

Exploring Frank's negative cognitions uncovered "I am unworthy," "I am unlovable," "I am insignificant." In order to further identify the source of his fears and insecurity, the Floatback technique brought up a Touchstone Memory from his early childhood. When Frank was five years old, without any prior warning or explanation his mother dropped him off at his grandparents' home. He didn't have any idea why he was there or how long he was staying. The image he had was his mother walking away from him as he stood on the porch with his grandmother. His mother didn't turn to say "good-bye" as she walked away or look at him as she drove off. He didn't see her again for five months. His negative cognition was "I am useless," which went along with feelings of anger, shame and powerlessness in his "gut."

Prior to being left at his grandparents' house, Frank's parents had divorced and his father had moved out. It felt unbearable to Frank to see his mother go away. For the first time, when reprocessing the memory of his mother leaving him on the porch, he spontaneously saw the anguish and fear on her face as she closed the car door and drove off. A flood of understanding and relief filled him as he finally realized that leaving him that day was not something his mother wanted to do. It was something she felt she had to do. Frank's acceptance and trust of other people, including himself, changed dramatically after this session. He was much more comfortable with himself and no longer felt the need to constantly please the ones he loved. With more processing, Frank's frequent headaches, forgetfulness, angry outbursts, irritability, sadness and feelings of insecurity disappeared. Now he could concentrate on losing the weight he'd accumulated by using food as comfort. That could help to get his diabetes, high blood pressure and chronic back pain under control.

Now, Frank's mother left him in good hands. His grandparents loved him. She was gone for a few months and then returned. He also may have been so upset when she left that he didn't remember her telling him why she was going or when she'd be back. He might have forgotten that, just as he'd forgotten the look on her face. But what actually happens is not as important as how it affects us at the time. At five years old, the situation caused Frank to be so upset that the experience was locked into his brain as an unprocessed memory. That memory held the emotions and physical sensations he had been feeling when she left. As children most often do, he blamed himself for her leaving. He believed that it was his fault. He then dealt with his fears of more abandonment by trying to please his grandparents so they wouldn't leave him too. Since they didn't go away, it reinforced his belief that he needed to please people for them to stay. When his mother came back, he kept up the pattern. And because she didn't leave again, in his mind it meant that he was right. That set the groundwork for the rest of his relationships.

Basically, the old emotions that he verbalized in his negative cognitions had been stored in his unprocessed memories from childhood. They ran him for the next 50 years and contributed to two divorces. His insecurity and anger drove everyone away. Then each failed relationship became stored in his memory networks in turn and reinforced his negative sense of himself as being unlovable, unworthy and insignificant. Many of his symptoms had been there for years. It was only the increase in headaches and desperate fear of losing his current wife that finally sent him into therapy. So, for each of us, the question becomes: How miserable do we need to be before we do something about it? If we recognize the problem is inside us, then we understand that we take ourselves wherever we go. That's the first step to doing something about it.

I'm Making Me Crazy

Processing doesn't only take place in a therapist's office. Many things can happen in our everyday lives that cause our emotions to change and insights to occur. While Ted needed therapy to process one set of memories, another set of connections came from reading a book. He wrote to me that when he decided to try therapy, *I was no more than a walking computer by this time, with little emotion left in my body. My hours were long, quite often extending to 18 hours a day. I held down three high-paying jobs and was bringing home $11,000 a month. I was grinding my teeth, and it was the pain from that problem that brought me first to my dentist, then to the TMJ clinic and finally to a psychologist.*

Ted had had a horrendous childhood with an extremely abusive father. He and his therapist targeted one of the pivotal Touchstone Memories and as Ted describes it, *I found it amazing that once each set was done, it became easier and easier to see that I was not to blame. I was only a child and I was totally innocent. I know my therapist had tried again and again to instill this thought in my head in other forms of therapy but it just wouldn't click in. This time with EMDR it worked, and I felt a great sense of relief that it was finally over.*

There was still much more EMDR work to do. However, one area of Ted's life changed just from understanding how he contributed to his own discomfort. While reading a chapter in one of my earlier books, he recognized that he reacted at work to someone he considered incompetent in exactly the same way as the person in the story, whose name was

"Jonas." That person had willingly offered his experience for the book in order to help others. Now Ted wants to do the same. As he puts it, *I discovered another problem resolved. It was the story of Jonas. As a district manager now, I have difficulties with some staff and this one hit the target. I could relate completely with Jonas and I even felt the words were exactly as I would have expressed them . . . the helplessness and lack of control.*

As I read slowly, I could feel the images of my assistant, Peggy, grating on me with her slowness and my helplessness to get her moving more quickly. And then the tables turned. As I read and thought of Peggy, I found the situation coming to life in the way it really was. Here Peggy was doing a task, and I was pulling her off in several different directions. It's no wonder the poor woman appeared so slow. I had her trying to do five different critical jobs in four different locations all at the same time. I had her running in circles and being pulled in several different directions. I started laughing so hard at the ridiculous scenario as I understood exactly what I was doing to her.

My stress was being caused by my own actions as a manager. I had her trying to do too much at one time. I've discovered a flaw in myself that I can now correct. I may be able to resolve four and five things at a time because I only have to work from my desk, but I can't ask a person to be in four or five places and attain that level of performance. I don't feel helpless anymore and I don't feel out of control. I feel I was the instigator in this issue. Peggy works much better now that I'm not breathing down her neck and trying to split her into several pieces so she can be faster and be in more places. I could see the original incident as to why this was happening—my father's demand for the impossible. I felt as out of control then as I did with Peggy. That is resolved now as well.

Like Ted, many of us may be run by unrealistic expectations of the way the world "should be." Often we don't realize that our standards and worldview are being dictated not by "reason," but by the unprocessed memories that are running our show. How much do our own control issues contribute to the stress in our lives? When we're stuck behind a slow driver on the highway, what do we do? If we can't find a way around, do we curse and stew, or are we able to let it go and enjoy our thoughts or the radio? If we can't let our frustration go, what purpose does it serve? Yes, people should know how to drive and either keep up with the speed limit or pull over. We may expect them to do that, but what if the slow drivers are preoccupied by the death of a loved one? What if they are elderly and haven't recognized they are in cognitive decline? What if they are simply self-absorbed people who think the world revolves around them? We have no idea what the reason might be. But clearly we're not being served by our stress. So can we take a moment to notice how we're feeling? Can we then commit to our own well-being and practice the self-control techniques to let go of our negative feelings? If not, maybe it would be worth using the Floatback technique when we get home to figure out why.

Staying Aware

Ted's experience is an example of why I've included so many stories in this book. I hope you've recognized yourself or a loved one or someone you are having difficulty with, and can now better understand what makes people tick. As Ted put it, he was planning to continue with his therapist in order to "use EMDR processing as the main weapon against the past." However, using the EMDR therapy techniques you've learned can give you an understanding of what is underlying your own issues, and sometimes that can be enough.

For instance, let's take the example of Joleen. She loved her husband dearly. So why had she been snapping at him for the past week, every time he asked her a question? Joleen and Alan had been together almost 30 years. They both felt they had found their soul mate and openly displayed their affection whenever they were together. But even though Joleen felt safe and content in Alan's arms, she noticed that something strange was happening. For no apparent reason, whenever Alan asked her a question she would bark at him impatiently. The feeling she had was of being relied on too much, and as the days progressed she felt more and more overwhelmed. She began noticing that whenever it happened she was left thinking, "It's all on me!" That made no sense since Alan shared equally in the chores and other day-to-day needs of a married couple. But as much as she breathed her way to calm after each incident, and often apologized, it kept happening.

In Chapter 1, I reminded you of the nursery rhyme, *Roses are red, Violets are blue.* Joleen was in a "Roses are red" phase. Roses are red— sometimes. So, since she had some important deadlines at work, Joleen brushed off her feelings at home, expecting them to go away. Maybe Alan asking a question was putting too much strain on her now, and her feelings were justified. Maybe. But then she noticed that along with the impatience, a despairing feeling that their marriage was over kept surfacing. Definitely, the feeling "It's over" was coming up—but that was nuts. Realizing that "Violets are NEVER blue," she finally took some action.

Using the Floatback technique on the words "I can't stand it. It's all on me" and concentrating on the feeling of being overwhelmed, she let her mind scan back. What popped up came with a head-slapping "Of course!" She was right back to last year, having returned to her childhood home, and was packing up her mother's belongings in order to move her to a nursing home. Her mother was in the hospital, and Joleen had rushed to her side from a business trip in order to take care of things. All the belongings needed to be in the nursing home before she left. Her brother lived nearby but fell ill and was unable to help. Joleen was forced to do it all alone. She'd spent a horrendous week pushing against her fatigue to complete the job.

By the time she left it was all done, but she was emotionally and physically exhausted. It was exactly a year since she'd finished the job and flown back home to Alan. Her mother never made it out of the hospital and died a couple of weeks later. No wonder Joleen was feeling "It's all on me" and "It's over." It was an "anniversary date" that may bring up negative feelings attached to a distressing event—sometimes year after year.

Joleen's realization of where the distress came from was enough to allow everything to click into place. The processing connections were made on the spot. The negative feelings disappeared, and Joleen stopped snapping at Alan. Life went back to normal. Sometimes that's all it takes.

PERSONAL EXPLORATION

One thing that Joleen had going for her was a daily practice of self-help techniques so that her general experience in life was calm and happy. That's why she was able to notice that something was wrong and do something about it. This brings us back to what you can choose to do in your daily life.

Daily Self-Care

For all of us, mental health has to be attended to in the same way we look after our physical health. Many studies have demonstrated the physical benefits of daily exercise (such as 30 minutes of walking 5 days a week) and of eating foods (such as cold-water fish and walnuts) or taking supplements that contain omega-3 fatty acids. These strategies are also useful for our mental health, as research has demonstrated how both can help relieve depression. In fact, in some studies a 30-minute physical workout 3 to 5 days a week over a 3-month period had the same effect as conventional antidepressants. Including both exercise and omega-3s as a part of your daily regimen can help make life easier, just as eating right and getting enough sleep are important for both physical and mental health.

The self-control techniques you've already learned should also be a daily practice. They will help you remain attuned to your own reactions. In this way you can more quickly recognize negative emotional states and can decide if they are getting out of hand—and what you need to do about it. Using the Safe/Calm Place, Spiral, Paint Can, Cartoon Character, Water Hose, Butterfly Hug (or alternate thigh tapping), Lightstream and breathing techniques can help get rid of disturbances when they arise. But it's important to practice and reinforce your arsenal of Safe/Calm Place techniques on a daily basis to make sure they stay strong enough to help you. I've included a *Personal Table* in Appendix A that you can copy and use as a checklist to keep yourself on track.

It's also important to keep up daily self-awareness practices in order to make sure that things haven't changed over time. Continuing with the TICES Log can help with that. It's possible that some personal qualities that allowed you to succeed at one stage of life can present problems later on. For instance, what you were able to accomplish easily at 20, 30 or 40 years old might take too much energy and physical exertion when you're 60 or 70. It's important to recognize physical limitations without feeling like a failure. But if you're being run by unprocessed memories, then the unconscious processes that previously helped to make you successful can now be debilitating. It doesn't serve you if memories that hold emotional states of "It's never enough; I have to succeed at all costs" push you beyond the capacity of your body. If you look carefully, you may find that an unprocessed "need to succeed" is taking too much out of you at any point in life. Why have inner turmoil to achieve success? Why not process the fears in order to succeed in peace? Other times new situations can upset us in ways that seem to make no sense at all. That's why a "Reevaluation Phase" is included in EMDR therapy in order to check how a person with newly processed memories is adjusting to the situation. For instance, Heather had negative beliefs from childhood of "I'm worthless" and "I can't succeed." At work she performed well enough to get by, but she was never able to deal with confrontation or stand up for herself. She and her therapist processed the associated negative memories, and she was now able to feel "I am good" and "I do have choices." Her behaviors at work changed and she was performing much better and was more assertive.

As her work improved, people began to notice and respond accordingly. For a while it felt good. But suddenly Heather found herself really upset because she had gotten a promotion. Why? This new positive feedback at work triggered an unprocessed memory with the emotions and negative belief of "If I'm too successful, I'll be abandoned." These associated fears had never been triggered before because Heather had not done very well previously. These fears came from an experience in school in which some of her classmates made fun of her when she got the highest grade on a book report. Once the underlying memories were processed, she was able to thoroughly enjoy her new success. Incidentally, many women can be burdened by that negative belief from misguided childhood warnings of "Don't be too smart or boys won't like you." It's common in many cultures.

It's important to remember that stress can come in many forms and from unsuspected places. Any of us can be negatively affected by stress— too many deadlines and not enough sleep can do it. Sometimes sudden crises can come up, and we feel temporarily overwhelmed. Our job is to stay aware of how we respond to life on a day-to-day basis and use our resources to keep from getting sucked into negative emotional states or beating up on ourselves because "It doesn't make sense." It actually does. It's simply cause and effect. Sometimes there is just too much going on and we're run-down. When that happens, we have to make other choices about our time and energy. However, when we're not making good choices, we need to remember to look within. What's preventing us from putting ourselves on the list of priorities? Is this a long-term pattern? If so, something needs to change. In determining what that is, remember that the perceptions of the outside world connect with and are colored by our memory networks. How we feel from moment to moment is influenced by what those memory networks contain. Whether it's our view of those around us or of ourselves, unprocessed memories may be running the show.

Developing a Timeline

If you've been keeping your TICES Log and using the Floatback technique along with the list of *Negative Cognitions*, then you should have a useful record of the current events that triggered you and the memories that go along with them. If you'd like, you can now start putting the memories on a *Timeline* so you can further understand your own history. Start a new section of your notebook and jot down the memories in the order of your age when they occurred. Start with the age, then the memory, the negative cognition and the SUD level. Skip a couple of lines between each entry. This will allow you to add any new Touchstone Memories if more get revealed over time as you encounter new challenging experiences or investigate other areas of your life. Once you've listed a memory on the *Timeline*, put a star next to it for every additional time you were affected by it. That will show you the ones that are really hot and generally running your show.

Take a minute and mentally check through your memories chronologically. On the *Timeline*, write down any other memories you consider the most disturbing from your childhood. For instance, is there a particularly troubling memory of your parents fighting or of your being ignored, humiliated or rejected? Bring it to mind. If you can feel it in your body at higher than a 4 SUD, then write down the number on the *Timeline*. Remember to use one of your self-control techniques to let go of any negative emotions after each one.

Now you can look over the *Timeline* to get a sense of when you developed different negative reactions, feelings and beliefs. It can also give you a good idea of which people in your life added to those problems. You might want to see whether any people you currently have difficulty with are similar to them. That should also help you recognize when you are being triggered in the present and remind you to do something about it. Using your daily care practice to self-monitor and to strengthen your self-control resources can increase your focus on well-being. That has important implications not only for you, but also for those around you.

FOUR ELEMENTS FOR STRESS REDUCTION

For all of us, stress can accumulate during the day. We can cope better with life when we take control of our own reactions, rather than having our overreactions control us. So we need to monitor ourselves and take steps to return to neutral when stress threatens to overwhelm us. Since many of us feel that going to work is like entering a war zone, I'm including a sequence of techniques that was initially designed for people living in areas affected by terrorist attacks. Because of the constant level of anxiety and high alert caused by the dangerous circumstances, the suggestions include reminders for daily use. I think the procedures are relevant to everyone living with high levels of stress.

Although we know it is important to self-monitor and use techniques when we find ourselves disturbed, sometimes we forget when we get stuck in a stressful routine. If you tend to get caught up in the demands, you can help yourself remember by wearing a colored bracelet or placing a sticker on your cell phone or computer or a picture on your desk. Whenever you notice it, check in to see how you are feeling. If you are feeling distressed, give it a SUD level. Then use the four techniques below until the SUD level decreases. The sequence of the *Four Elements: Earth-Air-Water-Fire* is designed to follow your body up from the feet to the head.

- *EARTH: GROUNDING, SAFETY in the PRESENT/REALITY:* Take a minute or two to "land" and to be here now. Place both feet on the ground and feel the chair supporting you. Look around and notice three new things. What do you see? What do you hear?

- *AIR: BREATHING for CENTERING:* You can use your favorite breathing exercise here. Another option is to breathe in through your nose as you count four seconds, then hold it for two, then breathe out for four seconds. Take about a dozen deep, slow breaths like this.

- *WATER: CALM and CONTROLLED to switch on the RELAXATION RESPONSE:* Check to see if you have saliva in your mouth. Make more saliva by moving your tongue around and imagining the taste of a lemon (or chocolate). When you are anxious or stressed, your mouth often "dries" because part of the stress emergency response involved in "fight or flight" shuts off the digestive system. So it seems that when you start making saliva, you switch on the digestive system again and the associated relaxation response. That's a theory used to explain why people are offered water or tea or chewing gum after a difficult experience. If you have difficulty making saliva, then start yourself off with a sip of water.

◆ *FIRE: LIGHT UP the path of your IMAGINATION:* Bring up the image of your *SAFE PLACE* or some other positive resource. Where do you feel it in your body?

As you combine all four elements, remind yourself that you can continue to feel the SECURITY NOW of your feet on the GROUND; feel CENTERED as you BREATHE in and out; feel CALM and in CONTROL as you produce more and more SALIVA; and you can let the FIRE LIGHT the path to your IMAGINATION to bring up an IMAGE of a place where you feel SAFE or a memory in which you felt good about yourself.

Remember that you now know a wide range of techniques to help control your stress levels. Many of us are so focused on our tasks at work or at home that we don't realize how much we are draining ourselves. We think, "Oh, I'll take care of myself later." But the effect of stress on our immune, cardiac and other bodily systems is both immediate and cumulative. It would be good to remember that life is a marathon, not a sprint. And it can be an enjoyable one at that.

FROM FAILURE TO FREEDOM

Many types of unprocessed experiences can hold us back from success in life. While some of them spring from childhood, problems can come from a wide variety of upbringings that on the surface may seem very different. For instance, Darlene came to treatment because of unbearable anxiety with her boss. Whenever she was the focus of his attention (whether positive or negative), she would blush uncontrollably, her skin would get clammy, and her heart would race. Her reactions were interfering badly with her work performance and putting her job at risk. In addition, she often experienced her boss as a "bully." He would sometimes yell at employees and shame them in front of others. He took no responsibility for his behavior. What bothered Darlene the most was her inability to "control my own body" even though intellectually she knew "he was a jerk."

The source of the problem came up during the Floatback. It turns out that Darlene's mother used to question her about all kinds of things. It seemed that she'd endlessly ask what Darlene had done during the day. Her mother wanted to know what other people said and did and just about everything Darlene thought and felt. The experience of being perpetually questioned felt invasive, out of control and irritating. But Darlene remembered feeling completely powerless to stop it. Her mother would keep going even when Darlene begged her to stop.

During processing Darlene began to sob, reporting that the worst part was the humiliation she felt. Often when they were in public situations, her mother would "remind her" of different things she had said over time and then "use it against her," embarrassing and shaming her in many different circumstances. At that point, Darlene exclaimed, "Wow, no wonder I'm so afraid when people start focusing their attention on me! It never made any sense to me why people paying 'good attention' to me would upset me so much. But now I'm realizing there was always a feeling of 'waiting for the other shoe to drop.' When were they going to embarrass me in some way? I can't believe THAT comes from THIS!"

While Darlene's anxiety came from a parent who was overly intrusive, Ryan had the opposite problem. As a child, he was pretty much ignored by his parents. He entered EMDR therapy because he felt paralyzed in making career choices. He was terrified of his boss' evaluation. Ryan always expected her to find errors in his work. Antidepressants hadn't helped, and his feelings were getting worse. This is an example where it becomes clear that being raised in the lap of luxury is no guarantee of mental health. Ryan's parents were wealthy and he was raised by servants. That led him to feel abandoned—that he wasn't worth his parents' attention. When he occasionally did spend time with his father, they'd play games that he was never allowed to win.

Not able to get his parents' positive attention led him to feel that he couldn't get what he wanted. As an adult, the negative cognitions that verbalized his emotional state were "I'm really no good. I can't be successful in my job." During processing, he described the physical sensation of a tightening in the pit of his stomach "like a rock." With further processing, the rock evolved into a smooth and warm presence, "like a foundation." Ryan called it "a strength and an example of soul." His positive cognition became "I'm capable of achieving on my own. I'll be OK."

The bottom line is that these early bedrock experiences from childhood can be the basis of what's holding you back in the present. However, with help they can be transformed into a newfound source of health. The causes of performance anxiety can run the gamut from some humiliation in a camp play, to never being able to please a parent, to something completely unexpected. For instance, Sean is a salesman who had the negative cognition "I'm not good enough" interwoven with an obsessive perfectionism. He had a feeling of anxiety before having to "perform"—whether for sales presentations or golf games. He knew his reaction was illogical. He had insight and skills to do well, but the high anxiety persisted and was harming his ability to succeed.

Focusing on his anxiety about a recent situation at work and the negative cognition "I'm not good enough," his clinician guided Sean in a Floatback technique. He then recalled a presentation in a drama class—along with the anxiety before and the relief he'd felt when it was over. During processing he remembered having received a standing ovation. Apparently, Sean's brain had stored the unprocessed memory of his performance without the information that he had done brilliantly. The processing led Sean to realize that he could handle any future events. Thinking of performing now produced excitement rather than anxiety and fear.

Self-Care

If you are anxious about making a presentation, you may be able to generate the shift from anxiety to excitement on your own. Many people believe it's necessary to feel anxiety because of misconceptions about how our bodies respond when presented with a challenge. Our brains prepare us for a challenge with a certain level of arousal. Performance research has indicated that there are optimal levels of arousal for different kinds of tasks. However, the way we view and deal with that feeling of arousal can make the difference between success and failure. In fact, some sports psychologists are now using the word "intensity" rather than arousal, anxiety or nervousness to eliminate the negative connotations people often have about these terms. Remember that there are many ways to feel the appropriate level of intensity, such as being excited by the thought of making a positive contribution.

Try concentrating on the positive aspects of what you are about to do. You can also manage the intensity of your arousal with your breathing techniques. At times, you can help shift yourself from anxiety to excitement by moving your mouth into a smile or changing your posture. Imagine a superhero giving the presentation. Allow yourself to step into the image and take that same stance. Just as people's shoulders sag and their postures collapse when they feel defeated, purposely bringing your shoulders back, straightening up, lifting your chin and smiling can help you shift out of anxiety.

In addition, take a look at the *Touchstone List* you made of recent events, memories and negative cognitions. Notice what negative cognitions get triggered for you. When it comes to job performance, is it "I'm a failure," "I'm not good enough," "I can't handle it" or "I can't make a mistake"? Take another look at the *Negative Cognitions* list to see which of them most connect with the feelings you are experiencing at work. Once you've identified the ones that come up for you, use the techniques you've learned to give yourself an alternative way to feel. Remember to develop and reinforce your Safe/Calm Place arsenal to include the positive emotional states you need to counter them.

Focus on your self-care. If you regularly feel "I'm not good enough," make sure to access daily the memories that allow you to feel worthwhile. If you often feel "I will fail," make sure to retrieve memories in which you succeeded. Savor those positive memories, feel the feelings, and let yourself enjoy them. Once again, concentrate on your body. Notice how you breathe, stand and hold your head when you bring up the positive memories. If you feel yourself getting triggered, try changing your breath and posture back to the way you feel in the positive states. Daily practice can help make the positive emotions, beliefs and body sensations more available to you when you need them.

LEARNING TO EXCEL

Most people would love to feel able to perform their tasks beautifully. But there is a big difference between doing something with confidence and inner peace, and being driven. For instance, Spencer is a middle-aged, divorced father of two sons working as a physical therapist. He came in for EMDR therapy on the recommendation of his girlfriend to treat his workaholism. He knew that his worrying about money and working too much were causing him to have angry outbursts. He recognized that as the reason his marriage had failed, and he didn't want his current relationship to break up. Spencer realized that his negative cognition "I have to be perfect" came from his father and grandfather. Their message to him was, "Work hard and do it perfectly." Processing included targeting a memory from the sixth grade when Spencer was studying math with his mother and had a tantrum because he couldn't understand the problems. He processed that successfully in one session and the positive belief that spontaneously arose was: "All I can do is the best I can and put everything else in perspective."

Centering Technique

Putting things into perspective includes the recognition that we don't need negative anxiety and fear to push us into top performance. We can simply enjoy what we're doing. Relaxation is a much better springboard than stress. In addition to your Safe/Calm Place arsenal and Breathing Shift technique, you can also use your breath for a Centering technique that many athletes, performers and executives have been taught to do.

There are many ways to "center" oneself. One of the best is to focus on your breathing. Read through the following paragraph and then give it a try.

> *Go inside and focus on your breathing. Be sure to breathe in S-L-O-W-L-Y through your nose. Notice the cool air as it enters your nostrils and hits the back of your throat. Imagine your windpipe as a glass tube that empties into your stomach. Notice how your stomach extends as you slowly breathe in. Notice the condensation of the warmed air on the glass tube as you exhale. Relax your jaw, exhaling through your mouth, and notice the drying of the warm air as it goes over your tongue and on the roof of your mouth. Repeat a few times and let the positive feelings build.*

Rehearsing for Success

Research has shown that mentally rehearsing a task before performing it can be extremely useful. For instance, visualizing successful free throw shooting prior to basketball games has been shown to improve performance, compared to games where only real-life physical practice was used. Even Olympic athletes use imagery exercises to fine-tune their responses. In fact, a survey conducted at a US Olympic athletic training center reported that 90% of the athletes used imagery to prepare for the competition. In addition, 94% of the Olympic coaches who were surveyed reported using imagery in their training programs. Personal coaches guide their clients in a wide range of professions to use imagery techniques. You can enhance your own performance at work or play by using your imagination in a focused way.

Research has shown that the same areas of the brain are activated when people are asked to remember doing something in the past and to imagine doing it in the future. As we've seen, if you have unprocessed memories from the past, they can color the way you view the present and the way you imagine acting in the future. Therefore, the full EMDR treatment includes three steps: processing the memories of the past that set the basis for the problems, processing the present triggers, and encoding new memories of success by imagining doing well in the future. During processing, disturbing memories transform into learning experiences that set the foundation for mental health. After processing, people automatically find themselves reacting to the world in new and positive ways. However, we use the third step, called a "Future Template," to help learn additional skills and further encode a pattern in the memory system for future success.

We generally do the steps in this order (past, present, future) because unprocessed memories can interfere with encoding new, positive ones. For instance, athletes may need to process memories of previous injuries and failures in order to deal with a lack of confidence, reduced motivation or performance anxiety. I've included some of the procedures for the Future Template here so you can use them at home. If no unprocessed memories are blocking you in this area, you can use this exercise to prepare yourself for challenges involved with future social situations or job interviews, or to fine-tune your business or athletic performance.

If there's a future situation that you would like help with, during the exercise you'll imagine yourself completing it happily and successfully. Even if you have difficulty imagining a successful resolution, the exercise will give you important information. If you hit any blocks, open your eyes and use one of your breathing techniques to return to neutral. Then try to identify any negative cognitions that may be there. Consider using the Affect Scan or Floatback technique to identify any unprocessed memories that may be interfering. See if there are any memories that should be added to your *Touchstone List*. If you are pushing against unprocessed memories, see if you can strengthen your Safe/Calm Place arsenal to help deal with them. If that doesn't work, consider having the memories processed with a therapist trained in EMDR.

First, identify the future situation you want to work on. Look at it realistically. Do you have the necessary information to succeed? If you have a test, have you studied? If you have to make a presentation, have you prepared the material? If you are performing, have you memorized your lines? If not, then your first task is to decide what prevented you from doing so. Imagining a success when you are not prepared with the basics is a real-life problem. If you have been procrastinating, then use the Floatback or Affect Scan technique to identify any unprocessed memory. Perhaps finding the source will help loosen its hold. Try using some of your self-control techniques to address any anxiety. Either way, it's important to complete your preparation before the real-life performance. You can also use the Future Template to imagine yourself completing the preparation successfully. Start by putting aside any distractions. Decide that you will deal with any intrusions after the exercise, and focus on the following steps.

Future Template

1. Relax your body and take several long, slow breaths. If you find your mind wandering, take another deep breath and bring it back to the exercise.

2. Focus on the future situation you'd like to deal with.

3. Decide how you would like to be seeing, feeling, acting and believing in that situation.

4. Use your Safe/Calm Place exercise to bring up the feeling you'd like to have by identifying some experience in your past where you succeeded.

5. Then bring up the positive cognition "I can succeed." Focus on the positive feelings, such as strength, clarity, confidence or calm.

6. Focus on an image of doing well in the future situation. Feel the positive emotions and body sensations that go along with it. You can enhance it even more if you let yourself get into it physically. Move yourself into the posture that allows you to feel successful and confident.

7. Run a movie in your mind of handling the situation well from start to finish. Make sure that the movie has a beginning, middle and end. Notice what you're seeing, thinking, feeling and experiencing in your body. Run the movie at least three times and enjoy the positive emotions and sensations.

8. Imagine some challenges arising, such as presentation equipment glitches, and imagine handling them with confidence and calm. Run that movie through to a successful conclusion.

Always make sure to end the sessions by returning to the positive imagery of your success. If any new challenges arise before your actual performance, you can run a new movie where you deal with the situation well. This helps set a memory pattern of success. If you find yourself disturbed during the actual situation, remember to use your self-control techniques. Anyone can get momentarily disturbed. Knowing how to deal with it is important for all successful executives, athletes and performers.

FROM SURVIVOR TO THRIVER

Therapy has sometimes been given a bad rap, as if it were somehow an indication of weakness. Personally, I consider it a sign of bravery. Millions of people have been wounded and yet they keep going—putting one foot in front of the other as they stay in relationships and jobs they hate. Often they do it for the best of reasons: I don't want to hurt anybody; I have a responsibility; I can't let people down. What therapy does for those who are brave enough to face their fears is to give them a new chance at life. A life where they count as much as the next person. Where "Love thy neighbor as thyself" means they can love themselves too. But you have to be willing to try. And if you are afraid to fail, that's coming from those memory networks that are pushing fears you didn't ask for and you didn't have the power to prevent when they were planted inside you. But you have the chance to let them go.

I also want to emphasize that it is your own brain doing the healing. If the brain's information processing system is stuck, you are simply getting assistance to give it a jump start. For instance, Jeanne came in because of anxiety related to an upcoming promotion. She would be supervising and routinely speaking to a group of 250 people. During the first history-taking session, she told her therapist, "There's nothing really big back there." So the therapist taught her the Safe Place technique and during the next session targeted Jeanne's anxiety and the feeling "I don't matter." They tried identifying a Touchstone Memory, but Jeanne insisted, "The feeling has always been there." So they focused on the first presentation she would have to do after the promotion. The negative cognition was "I don't matter" along with the emotions of fear and shame. It was pretty bad, with a 9 SUD and negative feelings in her throat and chest.

As her therapist guided the processing, Jeanne's mind could now make the appropriate connections. She saw herself at age three, sitting on her mom's lap and jabbering away. Then her stepfather came in, picked her up off her mom's lap, sat her on the floor and began to talk to his wife. Jeanne was right. The feeling of "I don't matter" had been there for a really long time. Then another memory came up when she was seven years old. Jeanne had just transferred to a new school in a new town and the kids on the playground told her she was fat and ugly. As the information from her adaptive memory networks connected, she realized that her stepfather was ignorant of parenting issues, and the children were just being typical kids picking on someone new. She was able to visualize herself at seven years old and realized how precious she was. She felt a parent's love as she embraced a new sense of herself. When that was complete, she and her therapist targeted the upcoming presentation and during the Future Template her positive cognition of "I matter" felt completely true.

They scheduled an appointment for the following week, but Jeanne called and cancelled. She said, "The presentation went great! I didn't have any problems at all. That was amazing! Thanks, I don't need to come in for the next session, but if I need you for anything in the future, I'll call."

The bottom line here is that therapists can be like coaches. They know how to help guide you so that the power of your own system can take over. Once it does, you can be off and running on your own. If unprocessed memories are blocking your ability to excel, then consider therapist assistance. The amount of time it takes depends upon the preparation needed for processing, the number of memories involved and how much "new learning" needs to take place. If you're interested in exploring the possibilities, you'll find resources and guidelines for choosing a therapist in Appendix B.

Remember that success in life is not just about alleviating stress and suffering. It's also about focusing on well-being in all areas of your existence. Negative unprocessed memories can be wrapping their tentacles around your life and pushing down your full potential. Identifying the areas where you are stuck and using the techniques you've learned can help you steer your life in the direction you'd like it to go. We all know that it's much easier to perform well when life is balanced and relatively free of anxiety and depression. Including the performance enhancement tools in this chapter is a logical step.

Work with elite athletes makes it clear that talent and ability are only a part of what it takes to perform well consistently. To stay motivated and manage stress and anxiety, some of the most relied-upon mental training techniques include the centering and imaging techniques you've just learned. Their effectiveness is not confined to only one area of success. For instance, Kyle was a top state-ranked high school athlete who came to therapy to work on his lack of confidence and motivation. He processed memories of injuries and distractions such as imposing opponents, parental comments and disappointing looks on his coach's face. A number of techniques, including those you've learned and a Future Template, were used to help him stay focused on the game. Upon graduation, Kyle received a scholarship to attend a prominent university as part of their NCAA Division I highly ranked team. As he said, "This doesn't just help with my sport, does it? I'm getting straight A's for the first time!" He'd attended an academically challenging parochial school and had been struggling with learning disabilities.

The bottom line is that you're never too young, or too old, to start taking control of your life.

BRINGING IT HOME

"I once was driving up a snowy hill in Spokane and my transmission slipped into neutral. The car in back of me swerved alongside, since I came to an immediate halt. When the driver got even with me he shook his fist, with an awful scowl on his face. As he pulled out in front, I saw his bumper sticker, which said, 'Visualize World Peace.' Where does it start? Or was it his wife's car?"

The quote above was part of an e-mail I received from a colleague about a year ago. It pretty well sums up the human condition. We strive to be one thing, and our emotions often just won't play along. Whatever names we may have for it, "higher/lower" or "light/darkness" play out inside all of us. We often just can't live up to who we want to be, and the world simply doesn't conform to the way we'd like to see it. So how we deal on a day-to-day basis is what ultimately determines how much happiness, and how much stress, we will have in our lives. That's where self-awareness and the commitment to mental and physical health come in.

We've already seen throughout this book how we can better understand who we are and what we can do about it. In this chapter, we'll explore how we can be influenced by our culture and society. In addition, we'll focus on some important challenges that each of us will have to face at some time or another. They offer more opportunities for self-exploration and can help explain problems that you and others in your life may be currently dealing with. I'll also give more suggestions for self-care that can open up new possibilities for personal well-being. What we choose to do in life has important consequences not only for ourselves, but also for others around us. Ultimately, we each may be more important than we think.

THE THREADS OF HUMANITY

In the first chapter of this book I said that as we look for answers, it's not about blame, it's about understanding. We can't blame ourselves for patterns that were locked in when we were youngsters. And although our parents helped shape who we are today, they too were shaped by their own life experiences. So while people are responsible for their own actions, we would often have to go back generations to fully understand our roots. In addition, we also may have "inherited" certain ways of looking at people that separate us from a sense of our common humanity. If we are trying to make the best choices for ourselves and our lives, it's good to look into all the potentially dark corners to see what might be hidden from our view.

Family Disconnections

All of us can in one way or another overcome our personal, familial and even social histories. We can move beyond these painful issues and embrace life fully without these old memories dragging us down. This was Helene's experience. Her life was a tangle of two stories—years of fiercely leaping obstacles peppered with bouts of self-destruction. She received a full scholarship to attend college, graduating with both a degree in sociology and a budding substance abuse problem. She went on to become a counselor for multihandicapped children during the day and a bartender and drug dealer at night. At age 27, she checked into a residential drug treatment center. Two friends had recently died violent deaths, one a suicide and the other a drug-related murder. She saw her own danger. It was only a matter of time before her drug-related activities would cause her to lose her job, her apartment, her freedom or her life.

After discharge from rehab she was able to stay clean, but suffered waves of depression and anxiety. She pushed through years of misdiagnosis, treatment failure and hopelessness, until she diagnosed herself with PTSD and, after doing some investigating, entered EMDR therapy. At that point she began to understand the source of her addiction. Growing up, Helene was often separated from her parents and sent away to live with her alcoholic relatives. It was during those periods that her Aunt Jan physically and sexually abused her and her other siblings. Everyone knew Jan was "terrorizing" the family, yet no one did anything about it. A heavy blanket of denial and silence covered the entire extended family. While it was extremely difficult, Helene addressed her pain from these experiences and was able to resolve her issues over the course of three years. Yet, five years later, she returned to therapy again, this time with a different goal.

While Helene was a productive and well-functioning person, she continued to have problems in one particular area. Ever since she completed her therapy, she was feeling alienated from her family since she was the only healthy, not-addicted-to-drugs-or-alcohol person in it. Why did her family seem doomed to extinction? She was watching the younger children going down the same path she had taken. What could she do about it? She also wanted to understand how some of her family members had become capable of such cruelty. As she researched their stories, Helene brought them to her therapist to act as a sounding board. Together they targeted the feelings that were stirred up. Helene felt pulled in two directions: She felt powerless to stop the family despair and she experienced "survivor guilt"—for "getting better" herself. She wanted a sense of peace and balance that she hoped would come with understanding her family's history and her current role within it.

She started with her maternal Aunt Jan, the woman who had done the most damage and the person Helene had lived with through much of her childhood. In studying Jan's history, she discovered a woman who had been born into the wrong culture at the wrong time. Her aunt was an outsider. She was a highly intelligent, noticeably masculine lesbian in a world that demanded her to be otherwise. All of the doors to the professions and lifestyle options she wanted seemed permanently locked to her. She lived with constant pressure from her family and culture to be someone she couldn't be. Undervalued and invisible, she simmered with a rage.

Clearly, having to live a lie can take a toll. But more factors have to be involved to turn pain to violence. For Jan, it was the abuse and neglect she experienced in her own childhood. Her father was unavailable, working 14-hour days, 6 days a week. Her mother couldn't cope with her children and often took out her frustration on Jan. Her mother, Helene's maternal grandmother, was a German immigrant who worked hard to blend into a culture that didn't welcome her. She was a woman of strong direction and intent, who felt compelled by her society to follow her husband's dreams instead of her own. She used alcohol to dull the pain, lashing out at her children when it wasn't enough. This all occurred during a time when the stigma toward female alcoholics was so strong that there were few treatment options available. Helene's Aunt Jan watched her mother slowly die of alcoholism, surrounded by family members paralyzed by secrecy and shame. Basically, Jan was raised by a drowning woman in a culture that didn't value or listen to women, in a time where differences were not tolerated, in a place where help seemed unavailable.

Helene found the same alcoholism and hopelessness in the family of her father. She learned that her paternal grandmother was Native American. She'd desperately hidden her heritage after many experiences with discrimination and racism. It was a "family secret" so deeply covered that Helene was never able to fully unearth all the details.

Probing her family tree helped Helene to more fully understand the sap that coursed through it for generations—a toxic substance called shame. She also found herself staring straight into the ugly faces of oppression: racism, homophobia and gender discrimination. Her story and the story of her family now made sense to her, and this knowledge helped her to move on. She ended this round of therapy realizing what she could do. She could set a good example for the children of her siblings by staying safe and sane herself, and by providing guidance/refuge to them when they needed it. She could also advocate for oppressed populations in her career.

As she put it: *It was only due to birth circumstances, skin color and other privileges that I had the opportunity to process and overcome my past. I saw the direction my pain was taking me. I broke the law, hurt myself and others, and experienced within me the potential to inflict much greater damage. Untreated pain begets more of the same. I am not OK with all of the details of my history, but I can move past it. I think I've deepened my understanding of my Aunt Jan's pain, but it will never be completely clear, as that is her story and I will never know all of it.*

I forgive my aunt and other family members, as it unhooks me, but forgiveness doesn't mean I welcome abusive people in my life. We all have choices in how we cope with our pain, and they could have managed theirs better. I now see my trauma as a result of generations of hatred, pain and misunderstanding, and that this is something much bigger than me and my family. I'm grateful I had the chance to get better, but it is not OK with me that others may not. It is not OK that throughout the world this type of pain keeps perpetuating itself, and I plan to do my small part to address this.

As each of us looks back on our own family history, I wonder how many will find people who have been abused, displaced or influenced by oppression, war or other forces out of their control. It helps to understand that these aren't just abstract concepts. They are experiences that helped forge our ancestors and who we are today. To this day, many people remain outcasts or the object of violence because of their gender, nationality, religion or sexual orientation. This leaves the question of what we can do in our own lives to overcome the destructive patterns in ourselves. Not only for ourselves, but also for future generations.

Sister/Brother or Other?

Those of us who have been bullied or excluded in school because we were different—short, tall, skinny, fat, wore glasses, were disabled, top or bottom of the class—understand how trapped and alone we can feel. The insults and humiliations can derail our feelings of confidence and cause us years of unending grief. Imagine how much worse it is when adults in power feel justified making negative comments because of the things that we allow to separate us—whether skin color, religion, gender or culture. Even though technology is bringing the world closer together, the daily news and the wars that seem endless continue to give us feelings of fear about the "other." This is another example of the solution being inside us, whether we've been on the giving or receiving end of it. The bottom line is that to help make the world a different place, the change has to start from within.

Kate was forced into therapy. She didn't want it, especially not from the short blond woman who walked through the door. What the heck did she think she could do for her? But Kate had no choice. She had been the manager of the department for the past 20 years and had received great reviews. She was the first African American promoted to that position. But now the central office of the multinational company was demanding that everyone in her position pass an exam that she'd already failed twice. The company had assigned this therapist to her and there was no way around it. She couldn't deal with the performance anxiety on her own, and if she refused this woman's help her boss would be furious. So she looked at Terry with resentment—but couldn't get out of it. Kate couldn't help making it clear that she felt stuck in the room with her, and she didn't like it.

Terry said she understood and sympathized. Then she explained that because time was short they would concentrate only on what might be keeping Kate from passing the exam. So after a quick preparation with a Safe Place exercise, Terry asked Kate to concentrate on the feelings of being "stuck in the room." After settling on a negative cognition of "I'm stuck" and the feelings of anger and resentment that went along with it, they began the processing. The theme quickly shifted to "I don't trust you!" Terry said, "Notice that" and with the next set of eye movements they were off and running. Up came images and scenes of all the prejudice Kate had endured. They kept traveling back in time and Kate didn't hesitate to verbalize her resentments. She was surprised at all the insults and obstacles she'd had to overcome to get to where she was today. She remembered a teacher who looked just like Terry putting her down. She told Terry, "You're just like her. I hate you." Now it made sense. Terry just said, "Notice that."

Kate remembered being called stupid and told that she'd never amount to anything—that she was only good enough to clean houses. The processing went on for the next five hours and by the end, her SUD was 0 and the positive cognition "I have choices" felt completely true. She realized that she could take the test that weekend even though she'd never been able to study properly or hold information before. She took the test and knew she'd failed it. But now it was different. She had no anxiety and confidently started to study for the next exam, which she passed. She also had no hesitation sending other personnel in the company to Terry for assistance. It felt to Kate that they were now two equals working together to help others.

Personal Exploration

The pain and resentment born of prejudice is always a two-way street. When we push others away or marginalize them, as a society we miss out on the positive contributions they could have made. As we react to people with fear and resentment, we breed it in others. The basic question is whether we want to be part of the solution or part of the problem. That means identifying the places where we're hurting—or hurting others. Consider looking for the resentment, fear, shame and pain you may be carrying and use the Floatback technique to identify where it's coming from. Use the self-control techniques you've learned to see if you can shift your reactions. Pain that has not been tended to can make you cruel, judgmental and abusive toward yourself and maybe toward others.

People who are secure aren't run by fear. They don't paint whole groups of people with one brush because one person from that group hurt them. Or because someone else said they should feel that way.

Remember that we are all vulnerable to the "horns effect." That's when we see one characteristic that we don't like and assume the person has a wide range of other negative qualities. It's the opposite of the "halo effect" where we assume a person has a variety of good qualities because we like one thing about them. Prejudice can put blinders on us so we can't see anything good about another person. In order to see others clearly, we need to be willing to see our own flaws as well so we can do something about them.

Most of us have heard the saying "Love your neighbor." But as families and individuals we can become increasingly isolated in our own communities. Maybe a good place to start is to just get to know others. This can help us all understand ourselves as part of the human family—a family that comes in a variety of shapes, colors, beliefs and lifestyle choices. Notice any fear or disdain of differences that might lurk inside of you and begin to gently ask some questions. Where did you learn it? Does it really serve you? What can you do to lessen it? Did your mistrust come from someone else's story, or were you personally hurt? If identifying where your feeling of separation or difference comes from doesn't help, does staying this way serve you? If not, consider processing the memory.

Ultimately, we have the freedom to choose. We are all like Kate, possibly singing someone else's song. The prejudice she'd experienced in her life separated her and made her just as judgmental about a person from another race as the ones that had been hurtful to her. By processing the memories, she dropped her anger and resentment toward others and got the poison out of her own system. That freed her to go further than she had ever gone before.

THE GREAT EQUALIZER

Regardless of how many issues divide us as human beings, many more things point to our similarities. And two challenges we all have in common are sickness and mortality. Each of us at some time or another will be faced with the loss of a loved one. How we deal with it is partially determined by our memory connections. For some, rather than mourning that eases over time, the grief will be complicated and remain intense because it is linking into unprocessed memories.

The World Is Gray

Jane was in her 50s and had lost her husband, Mike, about 6 months prior to coming in for therapy. She was functioning—working and handling her husband's business affairs—but internally she felt very stuck in the grief. She was depressed and all color seemed drained from her life. It wasn't getting any better over time. Everyone told her that it would become easier, but they'd been saying that for months and nothing had changed. She hadn't been able to cry, and things just felt bottled up. Her negative belief was "I'm powerless. I will never be able to move on."

Mike's death was targeted with EMDR therapy, and during the course of the reprocessing, Jane spontaneously thought about losing her mother to cancer as a young child. She remembered that before her death, her mother had said, "You must be strong." Both Jane and her mother knew she would die. This was a real "Aha!" moment for Jane. She realized she had taken her mother's directive very much to heart. She was just a young child—only nine years old—but she felt she had to be there for her father. Even after her mother's death, she didn't allow herself to grieve. She had pushed down any feelings of sadness and loss as signs of weakness.

Processing these memories freed up Jane to experience what she needed to feel. She recognized that her mother had not meant that she wasn't allowed to grieve. She'd just wanted her daughter to be OK. Jane suddenly had permission to let herself feel the emotions and go through the sadness stored inside her. As she told her therapist, "I can now grieve and move on." She understood that it was normal—it was all right to feel. She actively cried for Mike and, finally, for her mother. Feeling relieved and unburdened, she was able to continue moving through the grieving process gently, with positive memories of both her mother and husband that soothed her.

Many people in mourning have a sense of being stuck in the sadness, along with horrible images that continue to stab their heart. Particularly when someone dies suddenly, the person can be haunted by feelings of guilt as they think of all the things they "should have" said or done— and didn't when they had the chance. Those feelings of responsibility are often increased by images of their loved ones in pain. The memories often remain unprocessed and can cause grief to continue for years. For others, even if there is no guilt, there are only negative memories that keep feeding the sorrow. Happily, EMDR processing not only eliminates the intrusive negative associations, it allows the positive ones to return. For instance, two young brothers I treated only had negative memories of their father. He had been an alcoholic before he died and every time they thought of him, up came the images of him sitting in a ratty bathrobe surrounded by beer cans. Processing those memories allowed that picture to fade, and now when they thought of their father, up came memories of them all together on fishing and camping trips.

A study of EMDR therapy demonstrated that compared to another form of treatment, EMDR resulted in much greater recall of positive memories of the loved one, which came along with the sense of relief.

There are people who are stuck because they are afraid that by letting go of the pain of the loss, they will not honor the dead or no longer feel a connection. This simply isn't true. The emotional connections will be there without the pain. Just as any loved one would wish for you.

The World Is Black

While ongoing grief can poison our existence, for some the loss of a loved one can result in feelings of anger and the desire for revenge. This is particularly true when we lose someone to violence—and it has been feeding centuries of war in various countries. The pain moves from one generation to another, generating more and more violence. As we watch so many parts of the world in turmoil, we can support the humanitarian aid therapists who try to be part of the solution. For instance, a clinician in Pakistan has treated many who have survived acts of terrorism, as well as soldiers and aviation pilots who have been part of the "war on terror." He is sharing the story of his treatment of the children of a very high-ranking government official:

Their father fell martyr at the hands of a suicide bomber. His son and daughter were traumatized by the event as well as by the images of the body parts and blood of their father and his driver spread all over the road. The son wanted to leave his medical school and join a militant group to avenge his father's death. The daughter refused to leave her home and became mute.

Grief work and EMDR therapy over four weeks helped restore them and they both returned to their respective educational institutions. The daughter was married last year and is expecting a baby now. The son has completed his education and is now a doctor doing his internship in surgery. He wants to become a plastic surgeon. The two of them helped their family to launch a state-of-the-art secondary care hospital, built at their father's ancestral village. It is dedicated to the care of the families of survivors and martyrs of the war on terror. EMDR not only helped to alleviate their pain, agony and grief, but also led to positive outcomes in their personal lives. It helped them to transform their feelings of revenge into a meaningful and humanitarian pursuit.

This transformation of pain into the desire to help others is often a natural result of the healing process. It is a testimony to the potential we all have within us. Our information processing system is geared to allow us to learn what is useful and to let go of the rest. As we let go of the pain, we can be guided into a happy and productive future. And what is more useful than to help make the world a better place to live in for everyone?

Personal Exploration

Evaluate where you might be stuck in relation to someone who has died. Some of us have not been able to mourn or come to peace because earlier memories of pain keep a feeling of resentment alive after the person is long gone. For instance, Michelle entered therapy because of anxiety. Processing a current situation where she felt "stuck and helpless" brought up a memory of her father dangling her over a rushing river at age four. Since she was afraid of the water, he was trying to "desensitize" her by holding her there. It didn't work. What got locked into her memory network was the fear that if she moved to free herself, he would drop her in. The processing not only got rid of her "stuck and helpless" feeling—it spontaneously led to a healing reconciliation between Michelle and her deceased father.

It's never too late to make peace. So consider using a Floatback technique to help identify where you may be stuck in feelings of anger and resentment. What do you need to hold onto, and what can you let go?

MORE THAN ONE

As we've progressed through stories that show how unprocessed memories can affect our body, mind and emotions, we've seen how fear and a sense of powerlessness can often keep us captive. The same things that prevent progress in our personal development can also hold us back in what we can call "spiritual development." That is, a growth in understanding and a feeling of connection beyond our personal confines as mortals on this planet. In many traditions and religions, this translates to a sense of greater love and concern for humanity as a whole.

Sometimes these feelings of a greater spiritual connection are a natural outgrowth of processing. For instance, a woman who had been raped by her father many years ago was trapped in feelings of worthlessness. During the processing session with her therapist, her feelings shifted. At one point, after a set of eye movements, she said, "I just thought about love. 'God loves me' are actually the words that I thought!" She had a beautiful smile on her face and continued on the processing journey. She could not experience a sense of "God's love" until she was no longer trapped in her feelings of self-loathing. It was a spontaneous shift. For others, the blocks to this kind of greater inner peace may need to be addressed specifically.

Spiritual Disconnection

Some who strive for spiritual connections may find themselves blocked by unprocessed memories causing feelings of depression that prevent them from achieving their goals. For instance, Craig is a middle-aged man who came in for therapy complaining of fatigue, anger, poor sleep, feeling distant from his wife, and stress regarding a conflict with a former business partner. However, he spoke most about a disappointment with his spiritual journey and his practice of meditation for the past 30 years.

He chose his anger and disillusionment with meditating as his first target. Why couldn't he feel the sense of calm and peace that so many of his friends had during and after meditation? The feelings that continued to come up for him were "The world's not safe. Why engage in the world?" Craig and his therapist used the Floatback technique and up came the Touchstone event. He was three years old and had been knocked down by a neighbor's cow. Craig laughed out loud and shook his head as he recounted the story, saying, "It's a silly story but it still bothers me. The cow pushed me over with her nose and started licking my belly but I thought she was going to eat me. I called out for my mother. She didn't come for what seemed like a long time but was probably really only five minutes. What upset me most as a three-year-old was that my mother was laughing as she picked me up." That "misattunement" had locked in feelings of lack of safety and trust for more than 40 years. The positive cognition Craig started with was "I can handle it," but processing transformed it to "This is a building block for my strength." This was an important emotional realization in many ways. As with other memories that are keeping us stuck, the information processing allows a learning experience to take place so it becomes a foundation for our mental health.

At the next session Craig reported that he was sleeping better, was refocused on his spirituality, and had increased how much he exercised. He also reported that his anger had significantly diminished and he and his wife were communicating again. Then he processed another memory that related to the negative belief "The world's not safe. I can't deal with it." Craig was a teenager when he was carjacked, and his buddy was beaten up. He felt disgusted with himself for not fighting the thieves. This time the positive cognition was "I'm strong." At the next session Craig reported that his energy had returned and his sleep was fine. His meditations now connected him with a feeling of safety, peace and calm. He was also pleased that he spontaneously felt strong enough to handle and resolve the current conflict with his former business partner. Ultimately, there is no separation between body, mind, emotion and spirit. If unprocessed memories are blocking you in one area, they are likely affecting you in others as well.

The Seven Deadly Sins

Given that a goal of religion is to foster more meaningful connections with our inner world and with those around us, its tenets can also help to reveal where we may be blocked. Where do we strive and believe that we fail? For instance, Simon is a minister who wanted to use EMDR therapy to help him work on his spiritual development. From reading about the therapy and self-examination, he came to believe that "each of the Seven Deadly Sins is a trauma to our souls" that had originated from an earlier event in our lives. He felt that the sins he struggled with made him less effective as a husband, father and minister. And he believed that it was important to heal these sins within him.

Simon felt that he was lazy in taking care of chores at home as well as important tasks at church. Therefore, he chose to focus on Sloth. Simon's negative belief was "I say one thing then do another. I can't trust myself." A Floatback technique revealed that a Touchstone event had occurred when he was three years old taking a nap on the floor. His mother played an innocent game with him, saying, "It's time to get up from your nap." But when he tried to get up she would laughingly hold him back on the ground. Once this memory was reprocessed, Simon reported that he was more conscious of his actions and had more realistic expectations when choosing things to do. He was able to tackle bigger tasks at home and church, and handle them much more efficiently and less emotionally.

Wrath was another of Simon's targets. He reported that he had a long history of verbal outbursts and hitting the walls or doors at home when he was angry. This frightened his wife and daughter and he was ashamed of himself. The Touchstone event was observing his mother throw something at the kitchen clock when she was mad. He felt that gave him permission to explode whenever he got angry. The thought that went along with it was "If I explode in wrath, I have power and control." His desired positive cognition was "I am loving. I am a peacemaker." As the target was processed, Simon wept and said, "I want the courage to be authentic and vulnerable and have humility just like Christ during the crucifixion." By all reports Simon became more flexible, caring and loving to both his family and himself. He believes that by healing himself, he has become more complete as a person and a much better pastor. The bottom line is that if you are having difficulties living up to your own spiritual or religious beliefs, there may be unprocessed memories preventing it. You can do something about that.

The Final Doorway

While many of us find comfort in spiritual beliefs during our lives, often our greatest challenge comes when we are facing our own death. How we approach this final test of courage and strength is often based on how much fear is gripping us.

Two years following her diagnosis, the doctors told Donna there was nothing more to be done and that she should prepare for her passing. The cancer had taken over her body, yet it did not stop her desire to heal. She now turned inward to prepare herself for what was to come. She told her therapist that she wanted to clear up any further blocks inside herself so that she could "free her Spirit to move on." Although over the years she had continued to do her own inner work, she now said she wanted to find if there were any "leftovers."

Donna and her therapist began by establishing a Safe Place that she could use whenever she felt overwhelmed or the pain—physical or emotional—was too great. With her long-standing Catholic background, she chose to visualize herself next to Jesus with Mary's arm around her. At first, she began to cry and shake. As her therapist tapped her thighs, she took slow, deep breaths and said, "This is so comforting, I feel my whole body relaxing. There is a depth of comfort I have never experienced." Her body gently sank into the chair; even her feet relaxed. The ongoing tension in her face visibly softened.

The therapist asked her about the "leftovers" she'd mentioned before and if she was aware of anything that brought her discomfort. Donna looked up and said, "My father—I am afraid to see him after I die." From there they began to process her fear. She said, "I'm afraid he will be upset with me. I can feel it in my heart; it's heavy and it hurts." As they went through her thoughts and memories of her fear of disapproval, she ended by saying, "He has been with me all along, and he's proud of me. I can see his smiling face and my heart feels like it's opening."

Another "leftover" had to do with her feelings about the disease and her own responsibility in being sick. She wondered, "Did I bring this on? Is it my fault? Does anyone blame me?" She moved through feelings of anger at the cancer, the sense of betrayal about her body not being able to return to health, and self-doubt about whether she had fought hard enough. She ended with a deep sense of self-forgiveness and said, "I did everything I could, everything I knew to do at the time." She also said, with a sigh of relief, "Everyone in the family felt as helpless as I did; no one blames me."

As each day passed, Donna grew more tired and needed longer periods of rest. And each day the therapist visited her to continue to do the work together. Her family reported that she had gone from being highly agitated to more and more peaceful with less and less medication. Her pain was more manageable and when she was awake, she was more alert.

Donna focused on what would happen when she passed on. She visualized the "Pearly Gates." Her therapist asked, "How would you like it to go? Who will greet you?" She smiled and said, "I'm so light, moving is effortless, and yes he is there, my father, my mother and so many others that I love. I am smiling and so are they. There is no sadness and no pain. It's very bright and I feel like I lived a good life and I am moving on." After a period of silence she said, "This is a much easier move than the one I made as a child coming to this country, leaving my homeland and everything I knew. I was scared then. I'm not now." She was beaming during this processing. It was as if she was smiling from somewhere deep inside. In that moment, she had no awareness of her ravaged body. When her therapist asked her what she was noticing in her body, she said, "I feel light. I feel free! This is amazing!"

When Donna took her last breaths she had a gentle smile on her face. As her therapist said, "The Light of Life had always shone through her and now it had set her free."

Personal Exploration

Millions of people feel that faith is an important part of their lives and are comforted by prayer. Others believe in a higher power but feel separated and alone, unable to pray. Millions have sought inner peace through meditation, and many of them feel similarly blocked. In either instance, EMDR therapy can address these obstacles, which are often caused by unprocessed memories of pain, grief or disappointment. Once these barriers are removed, we are free to explore ways to deepen our spiritual connections through the practices that most resonate for us. This allows the choice to use prayer and meditation either separately or in combination to enhance daily life.

Clearly a person needs faith or spiritual beliefs to engage in prayer. But people only need to look at the science to have reasons to engage in meditation. Although in Western countries most people associate meditation with the Buddhist tradition, there are many forms that come from many different cultures. Recently some meditation practices have been separated from any particular belief system and evaluated in numerous studies. The research has documented that practicing these "focused attention" techniques can make it easier to handle stress and increases immune function. It's an excellent addition to daily self-care.

These meditation practices include "Mindfulness"—simply paying attention without attachment or judging. This is a part of the EMDR procedures, as the instructions during processing are to "Just notice." Rather than attempting to make something happen, just observe. While a clinician guides the client through the memory network to allow processing to occur, "just noticing" how your thoughts move can help you identify when you get stuck in a loop that doesn't get you anywhere. Sometimes this awareness alone can help loosen the memory's hold on you. People who meditate strengthen their emotional stability and the ability to stay mindful in daily life, allowing them to make better choices for themselves and for others.

Resources for guided visualization and meditation are in Appendix A. However, an easy way to begin is simply to sit quietly and notice your belly expand and contract as you breathe. Simply notice, quietly. If you find your mind drifting away to other things, then gently bring your attention back again to your belly. See if you can do it for five minutes at a time. Then increase your meditation time daily until you can sit comfortably for 20 to 30 minutes.

If you would like to also include your religious practices, consider adding a phrase from your orientation: "God is good" or "God is great" or "God is one." You could also use the word "Om" from the Indian tradition. Or a word such as "peace" or "love." Repeat the phrase or word each time you inhale and exhale. Also, meditation practices that focus on a sense of gratitude can be very helpful. Sit quietly and think of the things in your life that you are grateful for. Bring your attention to your heart and simply repeat, "Thank you for all you've given me" as you inhale and exhale. The "you" can be God or Spirit or Life or your own good nature.

These meditation practices can quiet both your mind and body, which can have valuable long-term physical and mental benefits. Also, importantly, they can remind you that you are more than any present disturbance in your life.

If you have previously felt spiritual connections but now feel blocked, this is another instance where unprocessed memories may be the cause. Sometimes the reasons may seem to be minor, as they were with Craig, whose Touchstone Memory was being licked by a cow when he was three years old. For others, the reasons may be a major trauma that has shaken their worldview. Those who have suddenly lost loved ones may feel separated and alone in unhealed grief. However, the processing of these memories can liberate the pain and return a sense of hope and connection. Even parents of children who lost their lives because of violence in the 9/11 attack, throughout the Middle East, or after natural disasters such as earthquakes, hurricanes and tsunamis can attest to a newfound sense of peace and reconciliation. We are all the same in our pain and in our ability to recover.

If you feel blocked but cannot think of a reason, then concentrate on the feelings you have in your body when you try to engage in prayer or meditation and use the Floatback technique to see if you can find a cause. If awareness itself is not enough to liberate you, consider having the event processed. The results may surprise you. Clinicians talk about a phenomenon called "posttraumatic growth." People who have been traumatized often report that recovery is more than just an elimination of pain. They can give positive answers to questions such as: What have I learned? How am I stronger? What am I grateful for? Who can I help because of what I know now? If something is blocked, perhaps it is time to let it be healed.

EMBRACING LIFE

As we've seen throughout this book, there are reasons for the reactions that we may have viewed as "crazy" or uncontrollable. Our unconscious memory connections are the foundation of our problems—and also our ability to find health and satisfaction in life. I hope that the stories and exercises have allowed you to see that you are not alone in either your pain or your desire for joy and well-being. Continuing to use the self-exploration procedures will increase your understanding about what's running your show. By practicing and using the self-control techniques on a daily basis, you can help increase your level of empowerment. If you seem blocked in any area, you also now know that there are options to allow you to move from feeling "stuck" into a life of new possibility and potential. Importantly, you now have the power to choose.

Another goal of this book is to help you feel greater compassion for yourself and for those around you. I hope you can feel compassion for both yourself as a child when your life's course was set—and for yourself as an adult who now has both the responsibility and ability to make needed changes. Also, I hope that you can look at others in your life and feel a similar sense of understanding for their struggles. They will need to make their own decisions, but just as Helene decided to do, perhaps you can provide a "guiding light" through your own healthy choices. Each of us by our actions creates a ripple effect that can have far-reaching consequences.

Over the past 20 years, more than 70,000 clinicians have been trained in EMDR therapy worldwide. During that time, EMDR associations have brought people together from all over the globe to share their stories and what they have learned. What has continued to warm my heart is that so many of the stories are ultimately tales of triumph. They provide examples of the resilience of the human spirit—the ability to come back from pain and adversity. Over and over they demonstrate the ability of people to express love under the most horrific circumstances. These stories show how people are able to overcome whatever obstacle life has thrown in their path.

Whether living in penthouses or mud huts, we are all bound more by our commonalities than our differences. We may believe that our religion or traditions or culture is superior to others. But the bottom line is that our brains, minds, bodies and spirits move to a common rhythm. What pains one would pain all. That's why I've felt honored to share some of these stories with you. After all, when we speak of "home," it is the place on this planet that we found ourselves in at birth and that helped forge our destiny. Even if we left our homeland, we carry the imprint of our family and place of origin within us. The beauty is finding that wherever we go, we all share the same physical systems—and a body, brain and unconscious that function in the same way. When we are cut, our bodies tend to heal unless there is a block. And what we've seen over and over again through EMDR therapy is that the information processing system of the brain is geared to do the same thing. Our pain can transform into something useful. We can choose the path we wish to take. And paths converge all over the world.

My Brother's Keeper

A few years ago Hurricane Paulina devastated a small Mexican town. A team of EMDR-Humanitarian Assistance Program (HAP) clinicians arrived to help those in need. As you know, the Butterfly Hug was originally developed to help do EMDR therapy with groups of traumatized children. The group protocol spread worldwide and has successfully treated children and adults after both natural and manmade disasters, including those on both sides of the Israeli/Palestinian conflict. Now it was time to help a new group of youngsters who were in pain. The children formed a circle, and the clinician asked them to do the Butterfly Hug as they processed their memory of the wind, rain and rushing water that had claimed so many lives.

Two brothers, 18 and 16 years old, were not involved in the exercise. However, they watched intently from a short distance away. After the exercise was finished, the younger boy, Carlos, approached the clinician to tell her their story and to ask how his brother Hector could do the Butterfly Hug with no arms.

Carlos said that the raging river had swept away all his family members one night during the hurricane. First the furiously rushing water had dragged away their parents as it destroyed their house. As the oldest brother, Hector had done everything he could to save all three siblings by holding them tight. But he was only able to rescue Carlos, because the water snatched the two younger children from his grasp. This effort had left Hector with enormous pain in both his arms as the two brothers huddled together alone, waiting for someone to come and help them. After two days the two boys were rescued. But when they finally managed to reach the hospital, Hector's arms were already gangrenous and had to be amputated.

The clinician asked Carlos to take her to his brother so she could show them how to do the Butterfly Hug. The clinician asked Carlos if he believed that his brother had done an enormous act of love to rescue him. He responded immediately and intensely with "Yes!" Then she asked him to place himself behind his brother, while Hector remained seated in a wheelchair. She directed Carlos to lean over so that one of his cheeks was in contact with Hector's cheek as he embraced his brother from behind. She then helped Carlos to cross his arms over Hector's chest.

Both boys breathed deeply as Carlos used his own arms to do the Butterfly Hug across Hector's chest. The clinician and the two boys together processed the traumatic memories. According to the clinician, "There are no words to express the transformation in the faces of the two boys from despair to deep love. It was the most beautiful sight I've ever seen."

Reaching Out

The willingness to reach out to comfort and care for others is another commonality that we share. When a mudslide washed away a village, it left 50 children as orphans. The EMDR-HAP clinicians came to help and used the group protocol. This time instead of the Butterfly Hug, they taught the children to do the bilateral stimulation through alternate thigh tapping. The next day, when they arrived to work again with the children, they found the group waiting for them. The children were tapping one another.

It seems clear that we, who have so much more power and resources than these children, can also reach out. We can reach out to help—and we can reach out for help. For each of us, our concerns may be different. For instance, what is home to you? Is it yourself, your family, neighborhood, country—or global community? Each needs our attention, and real change has to begin within those of us who know enough to care.

One of the experiences that touched me deeply happened at a training workshop about ten years ago. Clinicians had flown in from all directions to a small coastal town a week earlier. The night before they were to leave, everyone was feeling wonderful and so enthused and so happy in that beautiful environment that they went down to the beach. It was nighttime, but the stars were out and they wanted to swim in the cove as they'd done many times before. What they didn't know was that the tide had turned, and a rip current was passing through.

Smiling and laughing, a number of them walked into the ocean and started swimming but were caught in the current and were getting pulled away. A number managed to scramble to the shore and stood there together with others who hadn't gone in, watching the friends they had made, these other people, being drawn out to sea. They felt completely helpless and powerless to do anything about it. And those that were caught in the tide, in the ocean, were unable to get back. They felt completely alone and believed they were going to drown. We don't know who did it, but one person on shore said, "Let's link arms and form a chain." Then together they all walked very slowly into the ocean, sup-porting one another. They were able to reach each one, and pulled them all to shore.

That's what many people are trying to achieve worldwide through humanitarian assistance programs. To join with those who are willing to link arms, to help bring everyone back in, so that no one has to be out there alone drowning in the dark. So if you have an inclination in that direction, please consider joining forces to support the work—because there is so much that needs to be done. And we can do it with joy and gratitude for what we've been given in life. As one little ten-year-old girl said after processing her trauma, "Don't you just feel like you want to hug the whole world?"

ACKNOWLEDGMENTS

This book is the culmination of a decades-long journey made more joyous by the loving support of my wonderful husband, Bob Welch, and my dear friend and colleague Robbie Dunton. As for the creation of the book itself, let me begin with special thanks to Susan Golant for her light editorial hand and stellar assistance with many of the tasks needed to bring the volume to fruition. With gratitude to my Rodale editor, Shannon Welch, for her astute suggestions, and for carefully shepherding the book through the production process with the help of her talented staff members, Marie Crousillat and Amy King. Many thanks to my agent, Suzanne Gluck, for her invaluable guidance and support. Thanks also to Del Potter for his emergency computer rescue and tech assistance.

The writing of the book involved a wide circle of researchers and clinicians who deserve recognition for their many contributions over the past years. My appreciation to Robert Stickgold for his thoughtful publications on the relationship of EMDR, memory and REM sleep, and valuable suggestions regarding the neurobiology descriptions in this volume. Many thanks to Daniel Siegel for his valuable suggestions and pioneering work in the area of interpersonal neurobiology. I am grateful to Hope Payson, Deany Laliotis, Jennifer Lendl, Susan Brown, Tony Madrid and Ronald Ricci, who contributed detailed cases and were invaluable in framing the descriptions and recommendations in their specialty areas. Many thanks to Ad de Jongh, Steven Silver, Deb Wesselman, Lenore Walker and Julie Stowasser for sharing their expertise and suggestions as readers for specific chapters.

Additional appreciation goes to Deany Laliotis and to Patti Levin for their thoughtful clinical contributions in reading the entire manuscript at different stages of development. I am also grateful to Charlie Hitt, Robin Robbin, Jane Schuler-Repp, John Linderman, Brian Tippen and Christina Peterson, who read the chapters from a layperson's perspective to ensure that the book was "user friendly." In addition, I'd like to acknowledge the following innovators for their independent professional contributions: Cynthia Browning for the Floatback technique, Elan Shapiro for the Four Elements procedure, and Lucy Artigas and Ignacio Jarero for their development of the Butterfly Hug. My special personal thanks go to Stephen and Ondrea Levine for teaching me the Lightstream technique more than 30 years ago.

Over the past 25 years it has been my honor to be part of an ever-expanding group of clinicians and researchers who have dedicated their lives to the alleviation of human suffering. I asked some of them for assistance to help explain to the general public what we have learned about the brain's information processing mechanisms and "the fabric of the mind." They and their clients responded enthusiastically with examples from all parts of the globe. Reading the stories has given me great joy in seeing not only the universality of the human condition, but also how time after time the human spirit has triumphed in overcoming even the worst obstacles. I give my heartfelt thanks to those who contributed their stories. Whether or not they ended up in the book is only a reflection of the writing process itself—where one example naturally leads to another. But all served as wonderful inspiration for me, and touching reminders of why we do what we do. For that I am eternally grateful. Your names are listed on the next page. Please forgive me if I have missed anyone—and make sure to let me know.

George Abbot

Robbie Adler-Tapia

Katie Atherton

Uri Bergmann

Susan Brown

Cheryl Clayton

Susan Curry

Kathy Davis

Ad de Jongh

Lucina Artigas Diaz

Yulia Direzkia

Mark Dworkin

Nancy Errebo

Isabel Fernandez

Ellie Fields

Carol Forgash

Karen Forte

Sandra Foster

Wendy Freitag

Irene Geissel

Denise Gelinas

Sarah Gilman

Ana Gomez

Barb Hensley

Seema Hingorany

Arne Hofmann

E.C. Hurley

Mike Jameson

Ignacio Jarero

Ann Kafoury

Roy Kiessling

Dawne Kimbrall

Frankie Klaff

James Knipe

Nancy Knudsen

Cynthia Kong

Deborah Korn

Reni Kusumawardhani

Deany Laliotis

Ellen Latenstein

Roxann Lee

Jennifer Lendl

Patti Levin

Marilyn Luber

Tony Madrid

Jeff Magnavita

Stephen Marcus

Nancy Margulies

Jeri Marlowe

Priscilla Marquis

Helga Matthess

Therese McGoldrick

Christine McIlwain

Sushma Mehrotra

Liesbeth Mevissen

Edith Taber Moore

Joanne Morris-Smith

Katy Murray

Udi Oren

Elaine Ortman

Barbara Parrett

Hope Payson

Byron Perkins

A. J. Popky

Ann Potter

Jari Preston

Gerald Puk

Gary Quinn

Mowadat Rana

Ron Ricci

Maudie Richie

Gisela Roth

Curt Rouanzoin

Lynda Ruf

Mark Russell

Gary Scarborough

Zona Scheiner

Jens Schneider

Karen Schurmans

Carolyn Settle

Elan Shapiro

Valerie Sheehan

Jocelyn Shiromoto

Michel Silvestre

Greg Smith

Ute Sodemann

Roger Solomon

John Spector

Shinto Sukirna

Khadja Tahir

Rosalie Thomas

Laura Tofani

Linda Vanderlaan

Deb Wesselman

Kathleen Wheeler

Marshall Wilensky

Christine Wilson

Bennet Wolper

Janet Wright

Carol York

Mona Zaghrout

Al Zbik

APPENDIX A

Glossary and Self-Help Techniques

Affect Scan—Procedure using a current situation and body sensations to identify a Touchstone Memory. (Chapter 4, page 78)

Belly Breath—To help lower disturbance, inhale slowly and deeply while feeling your belly expand. Then slowly exhale as you feel your belly contract. (Chapter 5, page 118)

Body Changes—Change your posture or facial expression to move from anxiety to excitement or other positive emotional states. (Chapter 10, page 266)

Breathing Shift—Allows you to lower your distress level by changing your breathing pattern to one associated with a positive emotion. (Chapter 3, page 55)

Butterfly Hug—Bilateral stimulation with alternate shoulder pats that can be used to increase the safe/calm place, and for stress reduction. (Chapter 3, page 57; Chapter 6, page 148)

Cartoon Character—Allows you to deal with negative self-talk by making the critical voice sound comical. (Chapter 3, page 58)

Centering—Using deep and slow breathing to relax in a way taught to many athletes, performers and executives. (Chapter 10, page 267)

Floatback—Use current situation, negative cognition and body sensation to identify a Touchstone Memory. (Chapter 4, page 88)

Four Elements—A sequence of four stress-reduction techniques (Earth, Air, Water, Fire) to help deal with chronic stress, as well as a procedure to help in periodical self-monitoring. (Chapter 10, page 260)

Future Template—Using imagery techniques for skill building and peak performance. (Chapter 10, page 270)

Lightstream—Allows you to deal with unpleasant emotions by focusing on the physical sensations and "directing light" at the disturbance. Combined with the Safe/Calm Place technique, it may also be helpful to deal with insomnia. (Chapter 7, page 179)

Meditation—Mindfulness techniques to increase focus, concentration and positive emotional states. (Chapter 11, page 294)

Negative Cognitions—Negative beliefs that put into words the disturbing emotions and thoughts associated with the unprocessed memory. (Chapter 4, page 80)

Paint Can—Allows you to deal with an unpleasant mental image by "stirring the picture." (Chapter 4, page 80)

Relationship Suggestions—To help improve relationship communication, including the "I forgive you" technique. (Chapter 8, page 195)

Safe/Calm Place Arsenal—Allows you to bring up a wide range of positive emotions through different images or cue words. For instance, a feeling of calm connected to an image of being on a mountaintop or near an ocean. (Chapter 3, page 53; Chapter 5, page 106; Chapter 6, page 146)

Spiral—Allows you to deal with unpleasant feelings by "changing the direction" of the physical sensations. (Chapter 5, page 107)

Subjective Units of Distress (SUD) scale—Used to keep track of the intensity of distress associated with a current situation or old memory. From 0 (no disturbance) to 10 (worst distress imaginable). (Chapter 4, page 75)

TICES Log—A record to self-monitor daily disturbance. Lists the trigger, image, negative cognition, emotion, physical sensations and subjective units of distress (SUD) level. (Chapter 4, page 91)

Timeline—A list of Touchstone Memories, Negative Cognitions, SUD levels and age in the order in which the memories occurred that is created to better understand your history. (Chapter 10, page 259)

Touchstone List—A list of current disturbances and the earlier memories that set the foundation for the current reactions, along with age, SUD and negative cognitions. (Chapter 4, page 78)

Touchstone Memories—The earliest remembered events that may be causing current symptoms and problems. (Chapter 4, page 75)

Water Hose or Wet Eraser—Eliminate disturbing mental images by washing them away. (Chapter 3, page 59)

Guided Visualizations
and Meditation Audio Recordings

Available at the EMDR-Humanitarian Assistance Programs Web site: www.emdrhap.org/store/gv

Letting Go of Stress—by Emmett Miller, MD

Four guided relaxation techniques including the equivalent of a Safe/Calm Place exercise

Lightstream Technique—by Francine Shapiro, PhD

Guided visualization

Soft Belly Meditation—by Stephen Levine

Guided meditations

Personal Table

	Day/Date					
Used meditation/relaxation tape (20 minutes)						
Exercised (30 minutes)						
Reinforced Safe/Calm Place arsenal (10 minutes)						
TICES Log Used techniques to reestablish equilibrium (+/y, -/n, 0/not needed)						
Made positive contacts (family/friends)						
Had R & R (fun/relaxation—amount of time)						
Ate with awareness						
Had full night's sleep						
Do I have a sense of well-being?						
Evaluate last 24 hours (-10 to +10)						

Use this Personal Table on a daily basis to help keep yourself on track. As you evaluate each day, ask yourself: What could make it better? What do I need more or less of to live a more rewarding life? Do I need more relaxation time? More comfort with the self-help techniques? Do I have a sense of well-being? Or do I need professional assistance?

While personal problems and feelings of emotional distress may sometimes seem insurmountable, you do have choices. Remember to practice your self-control techniques and use your TICES Log to construct your

Touchstone List and Timeline. This will allow you to more easily see your patterns of response in daily living. They will also give you a better idea of the kinds of positive emotions and feelings you need to add to your Safe/Calm Place arsenal. In addition, if you choose to find a clinician for EMDR therapy, these practices will generally enable you to move more quickly through the history-taking and preparation phases of treatment. Personal therapy is a partnership with a responsible clinician. As one client put it: "My therapist is the banister on the stairs that I climb."

APPENDIX B

Choosing a Clinician

EMDR is a form of psychotherapy that is recognized worldwide as effective in the treatment of trauma and other disturbing life events. The eight phases of EMDR are designed to ensure that the client's emotions, thoughts and body reactions evolve into a healthy state (see www.emdria .org/8phases). There are numerous procedures for each phase and specialized protocols for different problems. The cases you have read in this book were provided by well-trained clinicians using the reprocessing procedures that have been tested and validated by research. It is important that the clinician you choose do the same.

It is important to make sure that your therapist has taken a course that is approved by the EMDR professional association in that region. The organizations starting on the next page maintain lists of therapists that you can use to find one in your area. It is important to check credentials, since some clinicians may have unknowingly taken substandard training. For instance, in the US some training is being offered that is only one-third the length of the approved courses.

EMDR should only be administered by a licensed (or supervised) clinician specifically trained in this form of therapy. Take time to interview prospective clinicians. Make sure that they have the appropriate training in EMDR (basic training is a minimum of six full days with additional supervision) and have kept up with the latest developments. As with any form of therapy, while training is mandatory, it is also important to evaluate other factors. Choose a clinician who is experienced with EMDR and has a good success rate. Make sure that the clinician is comfortable treating your particular problem. In addition, it is important that you feel a sense of trust and rapport with the clinician. Interview as many as you need to find one who is knowledgeable and feels right to you. Every treatment success is an interaction among clinician, client and therapy.

Ask:

1. Have you completed the training approved by the EMDR professional organization?

2. Have you kept informed of the latest protocols and developments?

3. Do you use the full eight phases as taught in approved trainings and validated by research?

4. How many people with my particular problem or disorder have you treated?

5. What is your success rate with other clients with these problems?

EMDR Therapy and Training Resources

EMDR Institute

The EMDR Institute has trained more than 60,000 clinicians in EMDR therapy since I founded it in 1990. It maintains an international directory of Institute-trained clinicians for client referrals, and trains only qualified mental health professionals according to the strictest professional standards. Trainings authorized by the Institute display the EMDR Institute logo. It is now one of many training organizations approved by EMDRIA.

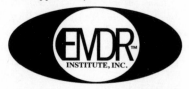

For further information on training or for a referral, the Institute can be reached by phone at (831) 761-1040, by fax at (831) 761-1204, by e-mail at inst@emdr.com, or by mail at PO Box 750, Watsonville, CA 95077 or visit the Web site at www.emdr.com

EMDR International Association (EMDRIA)

The EMDR International Association is a professional organization of EMDR-trained therapists and researchers devoted to promoting the highest possible standards of excellence and integrity in EMDR practice, research and education for the public good throughout the US. To identify a clinician near you who has been trained by an EMDRIA-Approved Basic Training Provider, visit their Web site and click on "Find an EMDR Therapist." If you are looking for a specific person who is not listed, then contact the organization by telephone or e-mail. Remember that many clinicians may not be aware that they have received substandard EMDR training.

For more information about EMDRIA, contact the association at:

5806 Mesa Drive, Suite 360, Austin, TX 78731–3785
Phone: (866) 451–5200 / Fax: (512) 451–5256
www.emdria.org or e-mail: info@emdria.org

EMDR CANADA is a sister organization in North America that maintains a list of trained therapists in Canada. Visit www.emdrcanada.org or e-mail info@emdrcanada.org

All of the multinational associations below perform a similar function to EMDRIA as the overseeing professional organization of their respective regions. They are devoted to promoting the highest possible standard of excellence and integrity in EMDR practice, research and education.

EMDR Asia Association

The EMDR Asia Association is the governing body for all the national EMDR associations throughout Asia, including Australia and New Zealand. Links to the individual national associations can be found on the Web site www.emdrasia.org or e-mail emdrasia@gmail.com

EMDR Europe Association

The EMDR Europe Association is the governing body for all the national European EMDR associations, including Israel and Turkey. Links to the individual national associations can be found on the Web site. Each national association maintains a list of members who have gone through the accredited trainings. Visit www.emdr-europe.org or e-mail info@emdr-europe.org

EMDR Iberoamerica Association

The EMDR Iberoamerica Association is the governing body for all the national EMDR associations throughout Latin America. Each national association maintains a list of members who have gone through the accredited trainings. Links to the individual national associations can be found on the Web site. Visit www.emdriberoamerica.org or e-mail info@emdriberoamerica.org

EMDRIA Latinamérica

Additional therapists are listed on their Web site www.emdr.org.ar

EMDR-Humanitarian Assistance Programs (HAP)

HAP, a 501(c)(3) nonprofit organization, is a global network of clinicians who travel anywhere there is a need to stop emotional suffering and prevent the psychological aftereffects of trauma and violence. The organization received the Sarah Haley Memorial Award for Clinical Excellence from the International Society for Traumatic Stress Studies in 2011. HAP's goal is to help break the cycle of suffering that ruins lives and devastates families.

The HAP model emphasizes training and giving professional support to local clinicians to continue the healing process. This training-focused model has several advantages. By teaching EMDR to local therapists, we are equipping them with an efficient and effective tool with which to treat the emotional effects of trauma. The professionals who are already part of the affected community are not being replaced by outsiders; rather, they are being given an important resource to be used when and how they think is best. Because reactions to traumatic events are sometimes delayed, and because individuals often try to resolve problems on their own before they seek professional intervention, training local clinicians helps ensure that when people do come for help, their needs can be met. In this way, effective psychological treatment of trauma extends far beyond the parameters of a single event.

HAP provides very low-cost EMDR training, in their own community, to therapists working in public and nonprofit agencies. US or international agencies that wish to sponsor such training should contact HAP directly.

In addition to training, **HAP's Trauma Recovery Network** coordinates clinicians to treat victims and emergency service workers after crises such as the Oklahoma City bombing and the 9/11 terrorist attacks.

Since the Oklahoma City bombing in 1995, a growing network of EMDR-HAP volunteers has responded to the calls for healing that come from all over the world, be it after Hurricane Katrina, severe flooding in

North Dakota, earthquakes in Turkey, India, China and Haiti, hurricanes or floods throughout Latin America, or volcanic explosions and tsunamis in Asia. We have reached out to communities traumatized by war and terror in Palestine and Israel, Croatia and Bosnia, Northern Ireland and Kenya, and to those weakened by epidemics in Ethiopia. We have helped to fill the void in mental health services for inner-city communities from Bedford-Stuyvesant to Oakland and for underserved populations in rural and suburban communities, Native American reservations, Hungary, Poland, China, South Africa, Ukraine, Mexico, Nicaragua, El Salvador and beyond. We have treated and trained and sowed the seeds for healing in the aftermaths of the TWA Flight 800 crash, the school shootings at Columbine High and Dunblane, Scotland, and the 9/11 terrorist attacks on New York and Washington.

EMDR-HAP volunteers typically donate at least one week per year of therapy or training time to make healing available to those who are suffering but who can least afford to pay for treatment. However, funding is required to get the clinicians to where they are most needed. While individual trainings in Asia, the Balkans and Africa have been cosponsored by organizations such as International Relief Teams and Catholic Relief Services, most are funded exclusively by individual contributions.

To learn more about HAP and what we have accomplished, visit www.emdrhap.org

Tax-deductible donations may be sent to:

EMDR-HAP
2911 Dixwell Avenue, Suite 201
Hamden, CT 06518
Phone: (203) 288–4450 / Fax: (203) 288–4060

APPENDIX C

EMDR: Trauma Research Findings and Further Reading

For an annotated list that includes more studies, see www.emdr.com/gpyp

Selected International Treatment Guidelines Designating EMDR Therapy as an Effective Trauma Treatment

American Psychiatric Association (2004). *Practice guideline for the treatment of patients with acute stress disorder and posttraumatic stress disorder.* Arlington, VA: American Psychiatric Association Practice Guidelines.

Bleich, A., Kotler, M., Kutz, I., & Shalev, A. (2002). A position paper of the (Israeli) National Council for Mental Health: Guidelines for the assessment and professional intervention with terror victims in the hospital and in the community. Jerusalem, Israel.

California Evidence-Based Clearinghouse for Child Welfare (2010). Trauma Treatment for Children. http://www.cebc4cw.org

CREST (2003). *The management of post traumatic stress disorder in adults.* A publication of the Clinical Resource Efficiency Support Team of the Northern Ireland Department of Health, Social Services and Public Safety, Belfast.

Department of Veterans Affairs & Department of Defense (2010). *VA/DoD clinical practice guideline for the management of post-traumatic stress.* Washington, DC: Veterans Health Administration, Department of Veterans Affairs and Health Affairs, Department of Defense. Office of Quality and Performance publication.

Dutch National Steering Committee Guidelines Mental Health Care (2003). *Multidisciplinary guideline for anxiety disorders.* Quality Institute Heath Care CBO/Trimbos Institute. Utrecht, Netherlands.

Foa, E. B., Keane, T. M., Friedman, M. J., & Cohen, J. A. (2009). *Effective treatments for PTSD: Practice guidelines of the International Society for Traumatic Stress Studies.* New York: Guilford Press.

INSERM (2004). *Psychotherapy: An evaluation of three approaches.* French National Institute of Health and Medical Research, Paris, France.

National Collaborating Centre for Mental Health (2005). *Posttraumatic stress disorder (PTSD): The management of adults and children in primary and secondary care.* London: National Institute for Clinical Excellence.

Randomized EMDR Trauma Studies

Abbasnejad, M., Mahani, K. N., & Zamyad, A. (2007). Efficacy of "eye movement desensitization and reprocessing" in reducing anxiety and unpleasant feelings due to earthquake experience. *Psychological Research, 9,* 104–17.

Ahmad A., Larsson B., & Sundelin-Wahlsten, V. (2007). EMDR treatment for children with PTSD: Results of a randomized controlled trial. *Nord J Psychiatry, 61,* 349–54.

Arabia, E., Manca, M. L., & Solomon, R. M. (2011). EMDR for survivors of life-threatening cardiac events: Results of a pilot study. *Journal of EMDR Practice and Research, 5*, 2–13.

Carlson, J., Chemtob, C. M., Rusnak, K., Hedlund, N. L., & Muraoka, M. Y. (1998). Eye movement desensitization and reprocessing (EMDR): Treatment for combat-related post-traumatic stress disorder. *Journal of Traumatic Stress, 11*, 3–24.

Chemtob, C. M., Nakashima, J., & Carlson, J. G. (2002). Brief-treatment for elementary school children with disaster-related PTSD: A field study. *Journal of Clinical Psychology, 58*, 99–112.

Cvetek, R. (2008). EMDR treatment of distressful experiences that fail to meet the criteria for PTSD. *Journal of EMDR Practice and Research, 2*, 2–14.

de Roos, C., et al. (2011). A randomised comparison of cognitive behavioural therapy (CBT) and eye movement desensitisation and reprocessing (EMDR) in disaster exposed children. *European Journal of Psychotraumatology, 2:* 5694 - doi: 10.3402/ejpt.v2i0.5694.

Edmond, T., Rubin, A., & Wambach, K. (1999). The effectiveness of EMDR with adult female survivors of childhood sexual abuse. *Social Work Research, 23*, 103–16.

Edmond, T., Sloan, L., & McCarty, D. (2004). Sexual abuse survivors' perceptions of the effectiveness of EMDR and eclectic therapy: A mixed-methods study. *Research on Social Work Practice, 14*, 259–72.

Hogberg, G., et al. (2007). On treatment with eye movement desensitization and reprocessing of chronic post-traumatic stress disorder in public transportation workers: A randomized controlled study. *Nordic Journal of Psychiatry, 61*, 54–61.

Ironson, G. I., Freund, B., Strauss, J. L., & Williams, J. (2002). Comparison of two treatments for traumatic stress: A community-based study of EMDR and prolonged exposure. *Journal of Clinical Psychology, 58*, 113–28.

Jaberghaderi, N., Greenwald, R., Rubin, A., Dolatabadim S., & Zand, S. O. (2004). A comparison of CBT and EMDR for sexually abused Iranian girls. *Clinical Psychology and Psychotherapy, 11*, 358–68.

Karatzias, A., Power, K., McGoldrick, T., Brown, K., Buchanan, R., Sharp, D., & Swanson, V. (2006). Predicting treatment outcome on three measures for post-traumatic stress disorder. *Eur Arch Psychiatry Clin Neuroscience, 20*, 1–7.

Kemp, M., Drummond, P., & McDermott, B. (2010). A wait-list controlled pilot study of eye movement desensitization and reprocessing (EMDR) for children with post-traumatic stress disorder (PTSD) symptoms from motor vehicle accidents. *Clinical Child Psychology and Psychiatry, 15*, 5–25.

Lee, C., Gavriel, H., Drummond, P., Richards, J., & Greenwald, R. (2002). Treatment of post-traumatic stress disorder: A comparison of stress inoculation training with prolonged exposure and eye movement desensitization and reprocessing. *Journal of Clinical Psychology, 58*, 1071–89.

Marcus, S., Marquis, P., & Sakai, C. (1997). Controlled study of treatment of PTSD using EMDR in an HMO setting. *Psychotherapy, 34*, 307–15.

Marcus, S., Marquis, P., & Sakai, C. (2004). Three- and 6-month follow-up of EMDR treatment of PTSD in an HMO setting. *International Journal of Stress Management, 11*, 195–208.

Nijdam, M.J. Gersons, B.P.R., Reitsma, J.B., de Jongh, A. & Olff, M. (2012). Brief eclectic psychotherapy v. eye movement desensitization and reprocessing therapy in the treatment of post-traumatic stress disorder: Randomized controlled trial. *British Journal of Psychiatry, 200*, 224–31.

Power, K. G., McGoldrick, T., Brown, K., et al. (2002). A controlled comparison of eye movement desensitization and reprocessing versus exposure plus cognitive restructuring versus waiting list in the treatment of post-traumatic stress disorder. *Journal of Clinical Psychology and Psychotherapy, 9,* 299–318.

Rothbaum, B. (1997). A controlled study of eye movement desensitization and reprocessing in the treatment of post-traumatic stress disordered sexual assault victims. *Bulletin of the Menninger Clinic, 61,* 317–34.

Rothbaum, B. O., Astin, M. C., & Marsteller, F. (2005). Prolonged exposure versus eye movement desensitization (EMDR) for PTSD rape victims. *Journal of Traumatic Stress, 18,* 607–16.

Scheck, M., Schaeffer, J. A., & Gillette, C. (1998). Brief psychological intervention with traumatized young women: The efficacy of eye movement desensitization and reprocessing. *Journal of Traumatic Stress, 11,* 25–44.

Shapiro, F. (1989). Efficacy of the eye movement desensitization procedure in the treatment of traumatic memories. *Journal of Traumatic Stress, 2,* 199–223.

Soberman, G. B., Greenwald, R., & Rule, D. L. (2002). A controlled study of eye movement desensitization and reprocessing (EMDR) for boys with conduct problems. *Journal of Aggression, Maltreatment, and Trauma, 6,* 217–236.

Taylor, S., et al. (2003). Comparative efficacy, speed, and adverse effects of three PTSD treatments: Exposure therapy, EMDR, and relaxation training. *Journal of Consulting and Clinical Psychology, 71,* 330–38.

Van der Kolk, B., Spinazzola, J., Blaustein, M., Hopper, J., Hopper, E., Korn, D., & Simpson, W. (2007). A randomized clinical trial of EMDR, fluoxetine and pill placebo in the treatment of PTSD: Treatment effects and long-term maintenance. *Journal of Clinical Psychiatry, 68,* 37–46.

Vaughan, K., Armstrong, M. F., Gold, R., O'Connor, N., Jenneke, W., & Tarrier, N. (1994). A trial of eye movement desensitization compared to image habituation training and applied muscle relaxation in post-traumatic stress disorder. *Journal of Behavior Therapy & Experimental Psychiatry, 25,* 283–91.

Wanders, F., Serra, M., & de Jongh, A. (2008). EMDR versus CBT for children with self-esteem and behavioral problems: A randomized controlled trial. *Journal of EMDR Practice and Research, 2,* 180–89.

Wilson, S., Becker, L. A., & Tinker, R. H. (1995). Eye movement desensitization and reprocessing (EMDR): Treatment for psychologically traumatized individuals. *Journal of Consulting and Clinical Psychology, 63,* 928–37.

Wilson, S., Becker, L. A., & Tinker, R. H. (1997). Fifteen-month follow-up of eye movement desensitization and reprocessing (EMDR) treatment of post-traumatic stress disorder and psychological trauma. *Journal of Consulting and Clinical Psychology, 65,* 1047–56.

Mechanism of Action

EMDR contains many procedures and elements that contribute to treatment effects. While the methodology used in EMDR has been extensively validated (see above), questions still remain regarding mechanism of action. However, since EMDR achieves clinical effects without the need for homework, or the prolonged focus used in exposure therapies, attention has been paid to the possible neurobiological processes that might be evoked. Although the eye movements (and other dual attention stimulation) comprise only one procedural element, this element has come under greatest scrutiny. Randomized controlled studies evaluating mechanism of action of the eye movement component follow this section. For an annotated list, see www.emdr.com/gpyp

Elofsson, U. O. E., von Scheele, B., Theorell, T., & Sondergaard, H. P. (2008). Physiological correlates of eye movement desensitization and reprocessing. *Journal of Anxiety Disorders, 22*, 622–34.

Kapoula, Z., Yang, Q., Bonnet, A., Bourtoire, P., & Sandretto, J. (2010). EMDR effects on pursuit eye movements. *PLoS ONE 5(5): e10762.* doi: 10.1371/journal.pone.0010762.

Lee, C. W., Taylor, G., & Drummond, P. D. (2006). The active ingredient in EMDR: Is it traditional exposure or dual focus of attention? *Clinical Psychology and Psychotherapy, 13*, 97–107.

Lilley, S. A., Andrade, J., Graham Turpin, G., Sabin-Farrell, R., & Holmes, E. A. (2009). Visuospatial working memory interference with recollections of trauma. *British Journal of Clinical Psychology, 48*, 309–21.

MacCulloch, M. J., & Feldman, P. (1996). Eye movement desensitization treatment utilizes the positive visceral element of the investigatory reflex to inhibit the memories of post-traumatic stress disorder: A theoretical analysis. *British Journal of Psychiatry, 169*, 571–79.

Propper, R., Pierce, J. P., Geisler, M. W., Christman, S. D., & Bellorado, N. (2007). Effect of bilateral eye movements on frontal interhemispheric gamma EEG coherence: Implications for EMDR therapy. *Journal of Nervous and Mental Disease, 195*, 785–88.

Rogers, S., & Silver, S. M. (2002). Is EMDR an exposure therapy? A review of trauma protocols. *Journal of Clinical Psychology, 58*, 43–59.

Rogers, S., Silver, S., Goss, J., Obenchain, J., Willis, A., & Whitney, R. (1999). A single session, controlled group study of flooding and eye movement desensitization and reprocessing in treating posttraumatic stress disorder among Vietnam war veterans: Preliminary data. *Journal of Anxiety Disorders, 13*, 119–30.

Sack, M., Hofmann, A., Wizelman, L., & Lempa, W. (2008). Psychophysiological changes during EMDR and treatment outcome. *Journal of EMDR Practice and Research, 2*, 239–46.

Sack, M., Lempa, W., Steinmetz, A., Lamprecht, F., & Hofmann, A. (2008). Alterations in autonomic tone during trauma exposure using eye movement desensitization and reprocessing (EMDR) — results of a preliminary investigation. *Journal of Anxiety Disorders, 22*, 1264–71.

Wilson, D., Silver, S. M., Covi, W., & Foster, S. (1996). Eye movement desensitization and reprocessing: Effectiveness and autonomic correlates. *Journal of Behaviour Therapy and Experimental Psychiatry, 27*, 219–29.

Randomized Studies of Hypotheses Regarding Eye Movements

Andrade, J., Kavanagh, D., & Baddeley, A. (1997). Eye-movements and visual imagery: A working memory approach to the treatment of post-traumatic stress disorder. *British Journal of Clinical Psychology, 36*, 209–23.

Barrowcliff, A. L., Gray, N. S., Freeman, T. C. A., & MacCulloch, M. J. (2004). Eye-movements reduce the vividness, emotional valence and electrodermal arousal associated with negative autobiographical memories. *Journal of Forensic Psychiatry and Psychology, 15,* 325–45.

Barrowcliff, A. L., Gray, N. S., MacCulloch, S., Freeman, T. C. A., & MacCulloch, M. J. (2003). Horizontal rhythmical eye-movements consistently diminish the arousal provoked by auditory stimuli. *British Journal of Clinical Psychology, 42,* 289–302.

Christman, S. D., Garvey, K. J., Propper, R. E., & Phaneuf, K. A. (2003). Bilateral eye movements enhance the retrieval of episodic memories. *Neuropsychology 17,* 221–29.

Engelhard, I. M., van den Hout, M. A., Janssen, W. C., & van der Beek, J. (2010). Eye movements reduce vividness and emotionality of "flashforwards." *Behaviour Research and Therapy, 48,* 442–47.

Engelhard, I. M., et al. (2011). Reducing vividness and emotional intensity of recurrent "flashforwards" by taxing working memory: An analogue study. *Journal of Anxiety Disorders, 25,* 599–603.

Gunter, R. W., & Bodner, G. E. (2008). How eye movements affect unpleasant memories: Support for a working-memory account. *Behaviour Research and Therapy 46,* 913–31.

Hornsveld, H. K., Landwehr, F., Stein, W., Stomp, M., Smeets, S., & van den Hout, M. A. (2010). Emotionality of loss-related memories is reduced after recall plus eye movements but not after recall plus music or recall only. *Journal of EMDR Practice and Research, 4,* 106–12.

Kavanagh, D. J., Freese, S., Andrade, J., & May, J. (2001). Effects of visuospatial tasks on desensitization to emotive memories. *British Journal of Clinical Psychology, 40,* 267–80.

Kuiken, D., Bears, M., Miall, D., & Smith, L. (2001–2002). Eye movement desensitization reprocessing facilitates attentional orienting. *Imagination, Cognition and Personality, 21, (1),* 3–20.

Kuiken, D., Chudleigh, M., & Racher, D. (2010). Bilateral eye movements, attentional flexibility and metaphor comprehension: The substrate of REM dreaming? *Dreaming, 20,* 227–47.

Lee, C. W., & Drummond, P. D. (2008). Effects of eye movement versus therapist instructions on the processing of distressing memories. *Journal of Anxiety Disorders, 22,* 801–8.

Maxfield, L., Melnyk, W. T., & Hayman, C. A. G. (2008). A working memory explanation for the effects of eye movements in EMDR. *Journal of EMDR Practice and Research, 2,* 247–61.

Parker, A., Buckley, S., & Dagnall, N. (2009). Reduced misinformation effects following saccadic bilateral eye movements. *Brain and Cognition, 69,* 89–97.

Parker, A., & Dagnall, N. (2007). Effects of bilateral eye movements on gist based false recognition in the DRM paradigm. *Brain and Cognition, 63,* 221–25.

Parker, A., Relph, S., & Dagnall, N. (2008). Effects of bilateral eye movement on retrieval of item, associative and contextual information. *Neuropsychology, 22,* 136–45.

Samara, Z., Bernet, M., Elzinga, B. M., Slagter, H. A., & Nieuwenhuis, S. (2011). Do horizontal saccadic eye movements increase interhemispheric coherence? Investigation of a hypothesized neural mechanism underlying EMDR. *Frontiers in Psychiatry* doi: 10.3389/fpsyt.2011.00004.

Schubert, S. J., Lee, C. W., & Drummond, P. D. (2011). The efficacy and psychophysiological correlates of dual-attention tasks in eye movement desensitization and reprocessing (EMDR). *Journal of Anxiety Disorders, 25,* 1–11.

Sharpley, C. F., Montgomery, I. M., & Scalzo, L. A. (1996). Comparative efficacy of EMDR and alternative procedures in reducing the vividness of mental images. *Scandinavian Journal of Behaviour Therapy, 25,* 37–42.

Van den Hout, M., Muris, P., Salemink, E., & Kindt, M. (2001). Autobiographical memories become less vivid and emotional after eye movements. *British Journal of Clinical Psychology, 40,* 121–30.

Additional Psychophysiological and Neurobiological Evaluations of EMDR Treatment

Bossini, L., Fagiolini, A., & Castrogiovanni, P. (2007). Neuroanatomical changes after EMDR in posttraumatic stress disorder. *Journal of Neuropsychiatry and Clinical Neuroscience, 19,* 457–58.

Kowal, J. A. (2005). QEEG analysis of treating PTSD and bulimia nervosa using EMDR. *Journal of Neurotherapy, 9(Part 4),* 114–15.

Lamprecht, F., Kohnke, C., Lempa, W., Sack, M., Matzke, M., & Munte, T. (2004). Event-related potentials and EMDR treatment of post-traumatic stress disorder. *Neuroscience Research, 49,* 267–72.

Lansing, K., Amen, D. G., Hanks, C., & Rudy, L. (2005). High resolution brain SPECT imaging and EMDR in police officers with PTSD. *Journal of Neuropsychiatry and Clinical Neurosciences, 17,* 526–32.

Levin, P., Lazrove, S., & van der Kolk, B. A. (1999). What psychological testing and neuroimaging tell us about the treatment of posttraumatic stress disorder (PTSD) by eye movement desensitization and reprocessing (EMDR). *Journal of Anxiety Disorders, 13,* 159–72.

Oh, D. H., & Choi, J. (2004). Changes in the regional cerebral perfusion after eye movement desensitization and reprocessing: A SPECT study of two cases. *Journal of EMDR Practice and Research, 1,* 24–30.

Ohtani, T., Matsuo, K., Kasai, K., Kato, T., & Kato, N. (2009). Hemodynamic responses of eye movement desensitization and reprocessing in posttraumatic stress disorder. *Neuroscience Research, 65,* 375–83.

Pagani, M. et al. (2012). Neurobiological correlates of EMDR monitoring—An EEG study. *PLoS ONE, 7(9)* e45753 doi:10.1371/journal.pone.0045753.

Propper, R., Pierce, J. P., Geisler, M. W., Christman, S. D., & Bellorado, N. (2007). Effect of bilateral eye movements on frontal interhemispheric gamma EEG coherence: Implications for EMDR therapy. *Journal of Nervous and Mental Disease, 195,* 785–88.

Richardson, R., Williams, S. R., Hepenstall, S., Gregory, L., McKie, S., & Corrigan, F. (2009). A single-case fMRI study EMDR treatment of a patient with posttraumatic stress disorder. *Journal of EMDR Practice and Research, 3,* 10–23.

Sack, M., Lempa, W., & Lemprecht, W. (2007). Assessment of psychophysiological stress reactions during a traumatic reminder in patients treated with EMDR. *Journal of EMDR Practice and Research, 1,* 15–23.

Sack, M., Nickel, L., Lempa, W., & Lamprecht, F. (2003). Psychophysiological regulation in patients suffering from PTSD: Changes after EMDR treatment. *Journal of Psychotraumatology and Psychological Medicine, 1,* 47–57. (German)

APPENDIX D

Selected References

This list provides selected references and suggested readings. Due to topic overlap, the lists for some chapters have been combined. Outcome studies relevant to the entire book appear in Appendix C. The full reference list for this book contains hundreds of additional citations and can be found at www.emdr.com/gpyp

Chapters 1 and 2

Trauma and EMDR

(For a more extensive list of controlled studies, see Appendix C.)

American Psychiatric Association (2004). Practice guideline for the treatment of patients with acute stress disorder and posttraumatic stress disorder. Arlington, VA: *American Psychiatric Association Practice Guidelines*.

Bisson, J., & Andrew, M. (2007). Psychological treatment of post-traumatic stress disorder (PTSD). *Cochrane Database of Systematic Reviews 2007*, Issue 3. Art. No.: CD003388. DOI: 10.1002/14651858.CD003388.pub3.

Bossini, L., Fagiolini, A., & Castrogiovanni, P. (2007). Neuroanatomical changes after EMDR in posttraumatic stress disorder. *Journal of Neuropsychiatry and Clinical Neuroscience, 19*, 457–58.

Department of Veterans Affairs & Department of Defense (2010). *VA/DoD clinical practice guideline for the management of post-traumatic stress.* Washington, DC: Veterans Health Administration, Department of Veterans Affairs and Health Affairs, Department of Defense. Office of Quality and Performance publication.

Lansing, K., Amen, D. G., Hanks, C., & Rudy, L. (2005). High resolution brain SPECT imaging and EMDR in police officers with PTSD. *Journal of Neuropsychiatry and Clinical Neurosciences, 17*, 526–32.

Levin, P., Lazrove, S., & van der Kolk, B. A. (1999). What psychological testing and neuroimaging tell us about the treatment of posttraumatic stress disorder (PTSD) by eye movement desensitization and reprocessing (EMDR). *Journal of Anxiety Disorders, 13*, 159–72.

Marcus, S., Marquis, P., & Sakai, C. (1997). Controlled study of treatment of PTSD using EMDR in an HMO setting. *Psychotherapy, 34*, 307–15.

National Collaborating Centre for Mental Health (2005). *Post traumatic stress disorder (PTSD): The management of adults and children in primary and secondary care.* London: National Institute for Clinical Excellence.

Ohtani, T., Matsuo, K., Kasai, K., Kato, T., & Kato, N. (2009). Hemodynamic responses of eye movement desensitization and reprocessing in posttraumatic stress disorder. *Neuroscience Research, 65*, 375–83.

Rodenburg, R., Benjamin, A., de Roos, C., Meijer, A. M., & Stams, G. J. (2009). Efficacy of EMDR in children: A meta-analysis. *Clinical Psychology Review, 29,* 599–606.

Rothbaum, B. (1997). A controlled study of eye movement desensitization and reprocessing in the treatment of post-traumatic stress disordered sexual assault victims. *Bulletin of the Menninger Clinic, 61,* 317–34.

Shapiro, F. (1989). Efficacy of the eye movement desensitization procedure in the treatment of traumatic memories. *Journal of Traumatic Stress, 2,* 199–223.

Shapiro, F. (2001). *Eye movement desensitization and reprocessing: Basic principles, protocols and procedures* (2nd ed.). New York: Guilford Press.

Wilson, S., Becker, L. A., & Tinker, R. H. (1997). Fifteen-month follow-up of eye movement desensitization and reprocessing (EMDR) treatment of post-traumatic stress disorder and psychological trauma. *Journal of Consulting and Clinical Psychology, 65,* 1047–56.

Stressful Life Events, PTSD and Other Symptoms

Arseneault, L., Cannon, M., Fisher, H. L., Polanczyk, G., Moffitt, T. E., & Caspi, A. (2011). Childhood trauma and children's emerging psychotic symptoms: A genetically sensitive longitudinal cohort study. *Am J Psychiatry, 168,* 65–72.

Bodkin, J. A., Pope, H. G., Detke, M. J., & Hudson, J. I. (2007). Is PTSD caused by traumatic stress? *Journal of Anxiety Disorders, 21,* 176–82.

Boyce, W. T., Essex, M. J., Alkon, A., Goldsmith, H. H., Kraemer, H. C., & Kupfer, D. J. (2006). Early father involvement moderates biobehavioral susceptibility to mental health problems in middle childhood. *Journal of the American Academy of Child & Adolescent Psychiatry, 45,* 1510–20.

Champagne, F. A. (2010). Early adversity and developmental outcomes: Interaction between genetics, epigenetics, and social experiences across the life span. *Perspectives on Psychological Science, 5,* 564–74.

Felitti, V. J., Anda, R. F., Nordenberg, D., Williamson, D. F., Spitz, A. M., Edwards, V., et al. (1998). Relationship of childhood abuse and household dysfunction to many of the leading causes of death in adults: The adverse childhood experiences (ACE) study. *American Journal of Preventive Medicine, 14,* 245–58.

Mol, S. S. L., Arntz, A., Metsemakers, J. F. M., Dinant, G., Vilters-Van Montfort, P. A. P., & Knottnerus, A. (2005). Symptoms of post-traumatic stress disorder after non-traumatic events: Evidence from an open population study. *British Journal of Psychiatry, 186,* 494–99.

Obradovic', J., Bush, N. R., Stamperdahl, J., Adler, N. E., & Boyce, W. T. (2010). Biological sensitivity to context: The interactive effects of stress reactivity and family adversity on socioemotional behavior and school readiness. *Child Development, 1,* 270–89.

Teicher, M. H., Samson, J. A., Sheu, Y-S, Polcari, A., & McGreenery, C. E. (2010). Hurtful words: Association of exposure to peer verbal abuse with elevated psychiatric symptom scores and corpus callosum abnormalities. *Am J Psychiatry, 167,* 1464–71.

Memory, Information Processing, Eye Movements and REM Sleep

(For an additional list of eye movement studies, see Appendix C.)

Duvari, S., & Nader, K. (2004). Characterization of fear memory reconsolidation. *Journal of Neuroscience. 24,* 9269–75.

Foa, E. B., Huppert, J. D., & Cahill, S. P. (2006). Emotional processing theory: An Update. In B. O. Rothbaum (Ed.), *Pathological anxiety: Emotional processing in etiology and treatment.* New York: Guilford.

Le Doux, J. (2002). *The synaptic self: How our brains become who we are.* New York: Penguin.

Llinas, R. R., & Ribary, U. (2001). Consciousness and the brain: The thalamo-cortical dialogue in health and disease. *Annals of the New York Academy of Sciences, 929,* 166–75.

Schubert, S. J., Lee, C. W., & Drummond, P. D. (2011). The efficacy and psychophysiological correlates of dual-attention tasks in eye movement desensitization and reprocessing (EMDR). *Journal of Anxiety Disorders, 25,* 1–11.

Shapiro, F. (2007). EMDR, adaptive information processing, and case conceptualization. *Journal of EMDR Practice and Research, 1,* 68–87.

Singer, W. (2001). Consciousness and the binding problem. *Annals of the New York Academy of Sciences, 929,* 123–46.

Stickgold, R. (2002). EMDR: A putative neurobiological mechanism of action. *Journal of Clinical Psychology, 58,* 61–75.

Stickgold, R. (2008). Sleep-dependent memory processing and EMDR action. *Journal of EMDR Practice and Research, 2,* 289–99.

Suzuki, A., et al. (2004). Memory reconsolidation and extinction have distinct temporal and biochemical signatures. *Journal of Neuroscience, 24,* 4787–95

Tronson, N. C., & Taylor, J. R. (2007). Molecular mechanisms of memory reconsolidation. *Nature, 8,* 262–75.

van der Kolk, B. A. (1996). Trauma and memory. In B. A. van der Kolk, A. C. McFarlane, & L. Weisaeth (Eds.), *Traumatic stress: The effects of overwhelming experience on mind, body, and society* (pp. 279–302). New York: Guilford Press.

Walker, M. P., & Stickgold, R. (2010). Overnight alchemy: Sleep-dependent memory evolution. *Nature Reviews Neuroscience, 11,* 218–19.

EMDR Session Transcript

Popky, A. J., & Levin, C. (1994). [Transcript of EMDR treatment session.] MRI EMDR Research Center, Palo Alto, CA.

The full session transcript can be found in:

Shapiro, F. (2002). Paradigms, processing and personality development in F. Shapiro (Ed.), *EMDR as an integrative psychotherapy approach: Experts of diverse orientations explore the paradigm prism.* Washington, D.C.: American Psychological Association Press.

Chapters 3 and 4

Different Therapy Approaches

Barlow, D. H. (Ed.) (2007). *Clinical handbook of psychological disorders, fourth edition: A step-by-step treatment manual.* New York: Guilford Press.

Cloitre, M., Cohen, L. R., & Koenen, K. C. (2006). *Treating survivors of childhood abuse: Psychotherapy for the interrupted life.* New York: Guilford Press.

Craske, M., Herman, D., & Vansteenwegen, D. (Eds.) (2006). *Fear and learning: From basic processes to clinical implications.* Washington, D.C.: APA Press.

Foa, E. B., Huppert, J. D., & Cahill, S. P. (2006). Emotional processing theory: An Update. In B. O. Rothbaum (Ed.), *Pathological anxiety: Emotional processing in etiology and treatment.* New York: Guilford.

Frederickson, J. (1999). *Psychodynamic psychotherapy: Learning to listen from multiple perspectives.* New York: Routledge.

McWilliams, N. (1999). Assessing pathogenic beliefs. In *Psychoanalytic case formulations.* New York: Guilford Press, 180–99.

Shapiro, F. (Ed.) (2002). *EMDR as an integrative psychotherapy approach: Experts of diverse orientations explore the paradigm prism.* Washington, D.C.: American Psychological Association Press.

Shapiro, F. (2001). *Eye movement desensitization and reprocessing: Basic principles, protocols and procedures* (2nd ed.). New York: Guilford Press.

Solomon, M. F., Neborsky, R. J., McCullough, L., Alpert, M., Shapiro, F., & Malan, D. (2001) *Short-term therapy for long-term change.* New York: Norton.

Weiner, I., & Craighead, W. E. (Eds.) (2010). *The Corsini encyclopedia of psychology* (4th ed.). Hoboken, NJ: Wiley.

Wolpe, J. (1990). *The practice of behavior therapy* (4th ed.). New York: Pergamon Press.

Genetics, Life Experiences and Psychological Problems

Arseneault, L., Cannon, M., Fisher, H. L., Polanczyk, G., Moffitt, T. E., & Caspi, A. (2011). Childhood trauma and children's emerging psychotic symptoms: A genetically sensitive longitudinal cohort study. *Am J Psychiatry, 168*, 65–72.

Brown, G. W. (1998). Genetic and population perspectives on life events and depression. *Soc Psychiatry Psychiatr Epidemiol. 33*, 363–72.

Boyce, W. T., Essex, M. J., Alkon, A., Goldsmith, H. H., Kraemer, H. C., & Kupfer, D. J. (2006). Early father involvement moderates biobehavioral susceptibility to mental health problems in middle childhood. *Journal of the American Academy of Child & Adolescent Psychiatry, 45*, 1510–20.

Caspi, A., Sugden, K., Moffitt, T. E., Taylor, A., Craig, I. W., Harrington, H., et al. (2003). Influence of life stress on depression: Moderation by a polymorphism in the 5-htt gene. *Science, 18*, 386–89.

Champagne, F. A. (2010). Early adversity and developmental outcomes: Interaction between genetics, epigenetics, and social experiences across the life span. *Perspectives on Psychological Science, 5*, 564–74.

Ellis, B. J., Essex, M. J., & Boyce, W. T. (2005). Biological sensitivity to context: I. An evolutionary-developmental theory of the origins and functions of stress reactivity, *Development and Psychopathology, 17*, 271–301.

Felitti, V. J., Anda, R. F., Nordenberg, D., Williamson, D. F., Spitz, A. M., Edwards, V., et al. (1998). Relationship of childhood abuse and household dysfunction to many of the leading causes of death in adults: The adverse childhood experiences (ACE) study. *American Journal of Preventive Medicine, 14*, 245–58.

Foa, E. B., Huppert, J. D., & Cahill, S. P. (2006). Emotional processing theory: An Update. In B. O. Rothbaum (Ed.), *Pathological anxiety: Emotional processing in etiology and treatment.* New York: Guilford.

Kendler, K. S. (1998). Major depression and the environment: A psychiatric genetic perspective. *Pharmacopsychiatry, 31*, 5–9.

Kendler, K. S., Hettema, J. M., et al. (2003). Life event dimensions of loss, humiliation, entrapment, and danger in the prediction of onsets of major depression and generalized anxiety. *Arch Gen Psychiatry, 60*, 789–96.

Luk, J. W., Wang, J., & Simon-Morton, B. G. (2010). Bullying victimization and substance use among U.S. adolescents: Mediation by depression. *Prevention Science. 11*, 355–59.

Meaney, M. J. (2001). Maternal care, gene expression, and the transmission of individual differences in stress reactivity across generations. *Annual Review of Neuroscience, 24*, 1161–92.

Obradovic´, J., Bush, N. R., Stamperdahl, J., Adler, N. E., & Boyce, W. T. (2010). Biological sensitivity to context: The interactive effects of stress reactivity and family adversity on socioemotional behavior and school readiness. *Child Development*, *81*, 270–89.

Pine, D. S., Cohen, P., Johnson, J. G., & Brook, J. S. (2002). Adolescent life events as predictors of adult depression. *J Affect Disord.*, *68*, 49–57.

Siegel, D. J. (1999). *The developing mind: Toward a neurobiology of interpersonal experience.* New York: Guilford Press.

van der Kolk, B. A. (1996). Trauma and memory. In B. A. van der Kolk, A. C. McFarlane, & L. Weisaeth (Eds.), *Traumatic stress: The effects of overwhelming experience on mind, body, and society* (pp. 279–302). New York: Guilford Press.

Butterfly Hug and Group EMDR Therapy

Fernandez, I., Gallinari, E., & Lorenzetti, A. (2004). A school-based EMDR intervention for children who witnessed the Pirelli building airplane crash in Milan, Italy. *Journal of Brief Therapy*, *2*, 129–136.

Jarero, I., Artigas, L., & Hartung, J. (2006). EMDR integrative group treatment protocol: A post-disaster trauma intervention for children and adults. *Traumatology*, *12*, 121–29.

Zaghrout-Hodali, M., Alissa, F., & Dodgson, P. W. (2008). Building resilience and dismantling fear: EMDR group protocol with children in an area of ongoing trauma. *Journal of EMDR Practice and Research*, *2*, 106–13.

EMDR Therapy Compared to Antidepressants

Van der Kolk, B., Spinazzola, J., Blaustein, M., Hopper, J., Hopper, E., Korn, D., & Simpson, W. (2007). A randomized clinical trial of EMDR, fluoxetine and pill placebo in the treatment of PTSD: Treatment effects and long-term maintenance. *Journal of Clinical Psychiatry*, *68*, 37–46.

EMDR Therapy for Combat Veterans

Carlson, J., Chemtob, C. M., Rusnak, K., Hedlund, N. L, & Muraoka, M. Y. (1998). Eye movement desensitization and reprocessing (EMDR): Treatment for combat-related post-traumatic stress disorder. *Journal of Traumatic Stress*, *11*, 3–24.

Silver, S. M., & Rogers, S. (2002). *Light in the heart of darkness: EMDR and the treatment of war and terrorism survivors.* New York: Norton.

Silver, S. M., Rogers, S., & Russell, M. C. (2008). Eye movement desensitization and reprocessing (EMDR) in the treatment of war veterans. *Journal of Clinical Psychology: In Session*, *64*, 947–57.

Chapters 5 and 6

Attachment, Parenting, Trauma and Neglect

Ainsworth, M. D. S. (1982). Attachment: Retrospect and prospect. In C. M. Parkes & J. Stevenson-Hinde (Eds.), *The place of attachment in human behavior* (pp. 3–29). New York: Tavistock Publications.

Bowlby, J. (1989). The role of attachment in personality development and psychopathology. In S. I. Greenspan & G. H. Pollack (Eds.), *The course of life: Vol. 1. Infancy* (pp. 119–136). Madison, CT: International Universities Press.

Dozier, M., Stovall, K. C., & Albus, K. E. (1999). Attachment and psychopathology in adulthood. In J. Cassidy & P. R. Shaver (Eds.), *Handbook of attachment: Theory, research, and clinical applications* (pp. 497–519). New York: Guilford Press.

Kennell, J. H., & Klaus, M. H. (1998). Bonding: Recent observations that alter perinatal care. *Pediatric Review, 19,* 4–12.

Klaus, M. H., Jerauld, R., Kreger, N., McAlpine, W., Steffa, M., & Kennell, J. H. (1972). Maternal attachment: Importance of the first post-partum days. *New England Journal of Medicine, 286,* 460–63.

Lyons-Ruth, K., Alpern, L., & Repacholi, L. (1993). Disorganized infant attachment classification and maternal psychosocial problems as predictors of hostile-aggressive behavior in the preschool classroom. *Child Development, 64,* 572–85.

Madrid, A. (2007). Repairing maternal-infant bonding failures. In F. Shapiro, F. Kaslow, & L. Maxfield (Eds.), *Handbook of EMDR and family therapy processes* (p. 131). New York: Wiley.

Main, M., & Hesse, E. (1990). Parents' unresolved traumatic experiences are related to infant disorganized attachment status: Is frightened and/or frightening parental behavior the linking mechanism? In M. Greenberg, D. Cichetti, & M. Cummings (Eds.), *Attachment in the preschool years* (pp.161–82). Chicago: University of Chicago Press.

Pietromonaco, P. R., Greenwood, D., & Barrett, L. F. (2004). Conflict in adult close relationships: An attachment perspective. In W. S. Rholes & J. A. Simpson (Eds.), *Adult attachment: Theory, research, and clinical implications* (pp. 267–299). New York: Guilford Press.

Porges, S. W. (2003). Social engagement and attachment: A phylogenetic perspective. *Ann NY Acad Sci, 1008,* 31–47.

Schore, A. (1994). *Affect regulation and the origin of the self: The neurobiology of emotional development.* Hillsdale, NY: Lawrence Erlbaum Associates.

Shapiro, F. (2007). EMDR and case conceptualization from an adaptive information processing perspective. In F. Shapiro, F. Kaslow, & L. Maxfield (Eds.), *Handbook of EMDR and family therapy processes.* New York: Wiley.

Shapiro, F., & Laliotis, D. (2011). EMDR and the adaptive information processing model: Integrative treatment and case conceptualization. *Clinical Social Work Journal. 39,* 91–200.

Shapiro, F., & Maxfield, L. (2002). EMDR: Information processing in the treatment of trauma. *In Session: Journal of Clinical Psychology, Special Issue: Treatment of PTSD, 58,* 933–46.

Siegel, D. J. (1999). *The developing mind: Toward a neurobiology of interpersonal experience.* New York: Guilford Press.

Siegel, D. J., & Hartzell, M. (2003). *Parenting from the inside out: How a deeper self-understanding can help you raise children who thrive.* New York: Tarcher/Penguin.

van Ijzendoorn, M. H. (1992). Intergenerational transmission of parenting: A review of studies in nonclinical populations. *Developmental Review, 12,* 76–99.

Waters, E., Merrick, S. K., Treboux, D., Crowell, J., & Albersheim, L. (2000). Attachment security in infancy and early adulthood: A twenty-year longitudinal study. *Child Development, 71,* 684–89.

Wesselmann, D. (2007). Treating attachment issues through EMDR and a family systems approach. In F. Shapiro, F. Kaslow, & L. Maxfield (Eds.), *Handbook of EMDR and family therapy processes.* New York: Wiley.

Memory, Perception and Trauma

Bower, G. H. (1981). Mood and memory. *American Psychologist, 36*, 129–48.

Heller, W., Etienne, H. A., & Miller, G. A. (1995). Patterns of perceptual asymmetry in depression and anxiety: Implications for neuropsychological models of emotion. *Journal of Abnormal Psychology, 104*, 327–33.

Herman, J. (1992). *Trauma and Recovery: The aftermath of violence–From domestic abuse to political terror.* New York: Basic Books.

van der Kolk, B. A., McFarlane, A., & Weisaeth, L. (1996). *Traumatic stress: The effects of overwhelming experience on mind, body, and society.* New York: Guilford Press.

Treatment of Phobias

Craske, M., Herman, D., & Vansteenwegen, D. (Eds.) (2006). *Fear and learning: From basic processes to clinical implications.* Washington, D.C.: APA Press.

Davey, G. C. L. (1997). *Phobias: A Handbook of theory, research and treatment.* New York: John Wiley and Sons.

De Jongh, A., & ten Broeke, E. (2007). Treatment of specific phobias with EMDR: Conceptualization and strategies for the selection of appropriate memories. *Journal of EMDR Practice and Research, 1*, 46–56.

Shapiro, F. (2001). *Eye movement desensitization and reprocessing: Basic principles, protocols, and procedures* (2nd edition). New York: Guilford Press.

Zimmar, G., Hersen, M., & Sledge, W. (Eds.) (2002). *Encyclopedia of psychotherapy.* New York: Academic Press.

Increased Reactivity to the Environment

Essex, M. J., Klein, M. H., Cho, E., & Kalin, N. H. (2002). Maternal stress beginning in infancy may sensitize children to later stress exposure: Effects on cortisol and behavior. *Biol Psychiatry, 52*, 776–84.

Meaney, M. J. (2001). Maternal care, gene expression, and the transmission of individual differences in stress reactivity across generations. *Annual Review of Neuroscience, 24*, 1161–92.

Obradovic´, J., Bush, N. R., Stamperdahl, J., Adler, N. E., & Boyce, W. T. (2010). Biological sensitivity to context: The interactive effects of stress reactivity and family adversity on socioemotional behavior and school readiness. *Child Development, 81*, 270–89.

Genetics, Life Experiences and Psychological Problems

See Chapters 3 and 4.

EMDR Treatment of Trauma

(For a more complete list of trauma studies, see Appendix C.)

Carlson, J., Chemtob, C. M., Rusnak, K., Hedlund, N. L., & Muraoka, M. Y. (1998). Eye movement desensitization and reprocessing (EMDR): Treatment for combat-related post-traumatic stress disorder. *Journal of Traumatic Stress, 11*, 3–24.

Edmond, T., Rubin, A., & Wambach, K. (1999). The effectiveness of EMDR with adult female survivors of childhood sexual abuse. *Social Work Research, 23*, 103–16.

Edmond, T., Sloan, L., & McCarty, D. (2004). Sexual abuse survivors' perceptions of the effectiveness of EMDR and eclectic therapy: A mixed-methods study. *Research on Social Work Practice, 14*, 259–72.

Rothbaum, B. (1997). A controlled study of eye movement desensitization and reprocessing in the treatment of post-traumatic stress disordered sexual assault victims. *Bulletin of the Menninger Clinic, 61,* 317–34.

Russell, M. C., Silver, S. M., Rogers, S., & Darnell, J. (2007). Responding to an identified need: A joint Department of Defense–Department of Veterans Affairs training program in eye movement desensitization and reprocessing (EMDR) for clinicians providing trauma services. *International Journal of Stress Management, 14,* 61–71.

Russell, M. C. (2008). War-related medically unexplained symptoms, prevalence, and treatment: Utilizing EMDR within the armed services. *Journal of EMDR Practice and Research, 2,* 212–26.

Silver, S. M., & Rogers, S. (2002). *Light in the heart of darkness: EMDR and the treatment of war and terrorism survivors.* New York: Norton.

Silver, S. M., Rogers, S., & Russell, M. C. (2008). Eye movement desensitization and reprocessing (EMDR) in the treatment of war veterans. *Journal of Clinical Psychology: In Session, 64,* 947–57.

Shapiro, F. (2001). *Eye movement desensitization and reprocessing: Basic principles, protocols, and procedures* (2nd edition). New York: Guilford Press.

Shapiro, F., & Maxfield, L. (2002). EMDR: Information processing in the treatment of trauma. *In Session: Journal of Clinical Psychology, Special Issue: Treatment of PTSD, 58,* 933–46.

Solomon, R., & Shapiro, F. (in press). EMDR and adaptive information processing: The development of resilience and coherence. In K. Gow & M. Celinski (Eds.), *Trauma: Recovering from deep wounds and exploring the potential for renewal.* New York: Nova Science Publishers.

Wesson, M., & Gould, M. (2009). Intervening early with EMDR on military operations: A case study. *Journal of EMDR Practice and Research, 3,* 91–97.

Chapter 7

Effects of Stress and Trauma on the Body

Altemus, M., Dhabhar, F. S., & Yang, R. (2006). Immune function in PTSD. *Ann. N.Y. Acad. Sci. 1071,* 167–83.

Arabia, E., Manca, M. L., & Solomon R. M. (2011). EMDR for survivors of life-threatening cardiac events: Results of a pilot study. *Journal of EMDR Research and Practice, 5,* 2–13.

Boynton-Jarrett, R., Rich-Edwards, J. W., Jun, H-J, Hibert, E. N., & Wright, R. J. (2010). Abuse in childhood and risk of uterine leiomyoma: The role of emotional support in biologic resilience. *Epidemiology, 9,* DOI: 10.1097/EDE.0b013e3181ffb172.

Chemtob, C. M., Nakashima, J., & Carlson, J. G. (2002). Brief-treatment for elementary school children with disaster-related PTSD: A field study. *Journal of Clinical Psychology, 58,* 99–112.

Cummings, N.A., & van den Bos, N. (1981). The twenty year Kaiser Permanente experience with psychotherapy and medical utilization: Implications of national health policy and national health insurance. *Health Policy Quarterly, 2,* 159–75.

Dew, M. A., Kormos, R. L., Roth, L. H., Murali, S., DiMartini, A., & Griffith, B. P. (1999). Early post-transplant medical compliance and mental health predict physical morbidity and mortality one to three years after heart transplantation. *Journal of Heart and Lung Transplantation, 18,* 549–62.

Grossarth-Maticek, R., & Eysenck, H. J. (1995). Self-regulation and mortality from cancer, coronary heart disease and other causes: A prospective study. *Personality and Individual Differences, 19*, 781–95.

Gupta, M., & Gupta, A. (2002). Use of eye movement desensitization and reprocessing (EMDR) in the treatment of dermatologic disorders. *Journal of Cutaneous Medicine and Surgery, 6*, 415–21.

Kelley, S. D. M., & Selim, B. (2007). Eye movement desensitization and reprocessing in the psychological treatment of trauma-based psychogenic non-epileptic seizures. *Clinical Psychology and Psychotherapy, 14*, 135.

Kusumowardhani, R. (2010). *Safe place and light stream stabilization techniques during the EMDR preparation phase are effective for coping with insomnia in women patients newly diagnosed with HIV.* Presentation at the EMDR-Asia Association Conference. Bali, Indonesia, July 2010.

Roelofs, K., & Spinhoven, P. (2007). Trauma and medically unexplained symptoms. *Clinical Psychology Review, 27*, 798–820.

Servan-Schreiber, D. (2004). *The Instinct to Heal: Curing stress, anxiety and depression without drugs and without talk therapy.* New York: Rodale.

Shapiro, F. (1989). Efficacy of the eye movement desensitization procedure in the treatment of traumatic memories. *Journal of Traumatic Stress, 2*, 199–223.

Shapiro, F. (2001). *Eye movement desensitization and reprocessing: Basic principles, protocols and procedures* (2nd ed.). New York: Guilford Press.

Shemesh, E., Yehuda, R., Milo, O., Dinur, I., Rudnick, A., Vered, Z., et al. (2004). Post-traumatic stress, nonadherence, and adverse outcome in survivors of a myocardial infarction. *Psychosomatic Medicine, 66*, 521–26.

Thombs, B. D., de Jonge, P., Coyne, J. C., Hooley, M. A., Frasure-Smith, N., Mitchell, A. J. et al. (2008). Depression screening and patient outcomes in cardiovascular care: A systematic review. *JAMA, 300*, 2161–71.

van der Kolk, B. A., McFarlane, A., & Weisaeth, L. (1996). *Traumatic stress: The effects of overwhelming experience on mind, body, and society.* New York: Guilford Press.

Panic Disorder

Craske, M. G., Roy-Byrne, P., Stein, M. B., Donald-Sherbourne, C., Bystritsky, A., Katon, W., et al. (2002). Treating panic disorder in primary care: A collaborative care intervention. *General Hospital Psychiatry, 24*, 148–55.

de Beurs, E., Balkom, A. J. L. M., Van Dijck, R., & Lange, A. (1999). Long-term outcome of pharmacological and psychological treatment for panic disorder with agoraphobia: A two year naturalistic follow-up. *Acta Psychiatrica Scandinavica, 99*, 59–67.

Fernandez, I., & Faretta, E. (2007). EMDR in the treatment of panic disorder with agoraphobia. *Clinical Case Studies, 6*, 44–63.

Feske, U., & Goldstein, A. (1997). Eye movement desensitization and reprocessing treatment for panic disorder: A controlled outcome and partial dismantling study. *Journal of Consulting and Clinical Psychology, 36*, 1026–35.

McNally, R. J., & Lukach, B. M. (1992). Are panic attacks traumatic stressors? *American Journal of Psychiatry, 149*, 824–26.

Oppenheimer, K., & Frey, J. (1993). Family transitions and developmental processes in panic disordered patients. *Family Process, 32*, 341–52.

Raskin, M., Peeke, H. V. S., Dikman, W., & Pinker, H. (1982). Panic and generalized anxiety disorders: Developmental antecedents and precipitants. *Archives of General Psychiatry, 39*, 687–89.

Childhood Asthma

Klaus, M. H., & Kennell, J. H. (1976). *Maternal-infant bonding.* New York: Mosby.

Madrid, A. (2007). Repairing maternal-infant bonding failures. In F. Shapiro, F. Kaslow, & L. Maxfield (Eds.), *Handbook of EMDR family therapy processes,* (pp. 131–45). New York: Wiley.

Madrid, A., & Pennington, D. (2000). Maternal-infant bonding and asthma. *Journal of Prenatal and Perinatal Psychology and Health, 14*, 279–89.

Suglia, S. F., Enlow, M. B., Kullowatz, A., & Wright, R. J. (2009). Maternal intimate partner violence and increased asthma incidence in children: Buffering effects of supportive caregiving. *Arch Pediatr Adolesc Med, 163*, 244–50.

Wright, R. J. (2007). Prenatal maternal stress and early caregiving experiences: Implications for childhood asthma risk. *Paediatr Perinat Epidemiol, 21(suppl 3)*, 8–14.

Wright, R. J., Cohen, S., Carey, V., Weiss, S., & Gold, D. (2002). Parental stress as a predictor of wheezing in infancy: A prospective birth-cohort study. *Am J Respir Crit Care Med., 165*, 358–65.

Phantom Limb and Other Pain

de Roos, C., et al. (2010). Treatment of chronic phantom limb pain (PLP) using a trauma-focused psychological approach. *Pain Research and Management, 15*, 65–71.

Flor, H. (2002). Phantom pain: Characteristics, causes and treatment. *Lancet Neurol, 1*, 182–89.

Grant, M., & Threlfo, C. (2002). EMDR in the treatment of chronic pain. *J Clin Psychol, 58*, 1505–20.

Halbert, J., Crotty, M., & Cameron, I. D. (2002). Evidence for optimal management of acute and chronic phantom pain: A systematic review, *Clin J Pain, 18*, 84–92.

Melzack, R. (1992). Phantom limbs, *Sci Am, 226*, 120–26.

Ramachandran, V. S., & Hirstein, W. (1998). The perception of phantom limbs, *Brain, 121*, 1603.

Ray, A. L., & Zbik, A. (2001). Cognitive behavioral therapies and beyond. In C. D. Tollison, J. R. Satterhwaite, & J. W. Tollison (Eds.), *Practical pain management,* 3rd ed. (pp. 189–208). Philadelphia: Lippincott.

Rome, H., & Rome, J. (2000). Limbically augmented pain syndrome (LAPS): Kindling, cortolimbic sensitization, and convergence of affective and sensory symptoms in chronic pain disorders. *Pain Med, 1*, 7–23.

Schneider, J., Hofmann, A., Rost, C., & Shapiro, F. (2008). EMDR in the treatment of chronic phantom limb pain. *Pain Medicine, 9*, 76–82.

Sherman, R. A. (1997). *Phantom pain.* New York: Plenum Press.

Body Image

Brown, K. W., McGoldrick, T., & Buchanan, R. (1997). Body dysmorphic disorder: Seven cases treated with eye movement desensitization and reprocessing. *Behavioural and Cognitive Psychotherapy, 25*, 203–7.

Buhlmann, U., Cook, L. M., Fama, J. M., & Wilhelm, S. (2007). Perceived teasing experiences in body dysmorphic disorder, *Body Image, 4*, 381–85.

Lochner, C., & Stein, D. J. (2003). Olfactory reference syndrome: Diagnostic criteria and differential diagnosis. *Journal of Postgraduate Medicine, 49*, 328–31.

McGoldrick, T., Begum, M., & Brown, K. W. (2008). EMDR and olfactory reference syndrome: A case series. *Journal of EMDR Practice and Research, 2,* 63–68.

Osman, S., Cooper, M., Hackmann, A., & Veale, D. (2004). Spontaneously occurring images and early memories in people with body dysmorphic disorder. *Memory, 12,* 428–36.

Phillips, K. A. (1991). Body dysmorphic disorder: The distress of imagined ugliness. *American Journal of Psychiatry, 148,* 1138–49.

ADHD and Intellectual Disability

Barol, B. I., & Seubert, A. (2010). Stepping stones: EMDR treatment of individuals with intellectual and developmental disabilities and challenging behavior. *Journal of EMDR Practice and Research, 4,* 156–69.

Evans, W. N., Morrill, M. S., & Parente, S. T. (2010). Measuring inappropriate medical diagnosis and treatment in survey data: The case of ADHD among school-age children. *Journal of Health Economics, 29,* 657–73.

Faraone, S. V., & Mick, E. (2010). Molecular genetics of attention deficit hyperactivity disorder. *Psychiatric Clinics of North America, 33,* 159–80.

Mayes, S. D., Calhoun, S. L., & Crowell, E. W. (2000). Learning disabilities and ADHD: Overlapping spectrum disorders. *Journal of Learning Disabilities, 33,* 417–24.

Mevissen, L., Lievegoed, R., & De Jongh, A. (2010). EMDR treatment in people with mild ID and PTSD: 4 cases. *Psychiatric Quarterly* , DOI: 10.1007/s11126-010-9147-x.

Visser, S. N., Lesesne, C. A., & Perou, R. (2007). National estimates and factors associated with medication treatment for childhood attention-deficit/hyperactivity disorder. *Pediatrics, 119* (Supplement 1), S99–S109.

Zuvekas, S. H., Vitiello, B., & Norquist, G. S. (2006). Recent trends in stimulant medication use among U.S. children. *American Journal of Psychiatry, 163,* 579–85.

Chapter 8

Overview of Family Therapies

Bowen, M. (1978). *Family Therapy in Clinical Practice.* New York: Aronson.

Kaslow, F. (2007). Family systems theories and therapeutic applications: A contextual overview. In F. Shapiro, F. Kaslow, & L. Maxfield (Eds.), *Handbook of EMDR and family therapy processes (pp. 35–75).* New York: Wiley.

Attachment and Adult Relationships

Banse, R. (2004). Adult attachment and marital satisfaction: Evidence for dyadic configuration effects. *Journal of Social and Personal Relationships, 21,* 273–82.

Davila, J. (2003). Attachment processes in couple therapy. In S. Johnson & V. Whiffen (Eds.), *Attachment processes in couples and family therapy* (pp. 124–43). New York: Guilford Press.

Johnson, S., & Whiffen, V. (2003). *Attachment processes in couples and family therapy.* New York: Guilford Press.

Treatment of Family Problems

Adler-Tapia, R., Settle, C., & Shapiro, F. (2012). Eye movement desensitization and reprocessing (EMDR) psychotherapy with children who have experienced sexual abuse and trauma. In P. Goodyear-Brown (Ed.), *The handbook of child sexual abuse: Identification, assessment and treatment.* (pp. 229–50) Hoboken, NJ: Wiley.

Bardin, A. (2004). EMDR within a family system. *Journal of Family Psychology, 15,* 47–61.

Brown, S., & Shapiro, F. (2006). EMDR in the treatment of borderline personality disorder. *Clinical Case Studies, 5,* 403–20.

Errebo, N., & Sommers-Flanagan, R. (2007). EMDR and emotionally focused couple therapy for war veteran couples. In F. Shapiro, F. Kaslow, & L. Maxfield (Eds.), *Handbook of EMDR and family therapy processes* (pp. 202–22). New York: Wiley.

Knudsen, N. (2007). Integrating EMDR and Bowen Theory in treating chronic relationship dysfunction. In F. Shapiro, F. Kaslow, & L. Maxfield (Eds.), *Handbook of EMDR and family therapy processes* (pp. 169–86). New York: Wiley.

Shapiro, F. (2001). *Eye movement desensitization and reprocessing: Basic principles, protocols, and procedures* (2nd edition). New York: Guilford Press.

Stowasser, J. (2007). EMDR and family therapy in the treatment of domestic violence. In F. Shapiro, F. Kaslow, & L. Maxfield (Eds.), *Handbook of EMDR and family Therapy Processes* (pp. 243–61). New York: Wiley.

Tofani, L. R. (2007). Complex separation, individuation processes, and anxiety disorders in young adulthood. In F. Shapiro, F. Kaslow, & L. Maxfield (Eds.), *Handbook of EMDR and family therapy processes* (pp. 265–68). New York: Wiley.

Wesselmann, D. (2007). Treating attachment issues through EMDR and a family systems approach. In F. Shapiro, F. Kaslow, & L. Maxfield (Eds.), *Handbook of EMDR and family therapy processes* (pp. 113–30). New York: Wiley.

Domestic Abuse

Burke, J. G., Lee, L. C., & O'Campo, P. (2008). An exploration of maternal intimate partner violence experiences and infant general health and temperament. *Maternal Child Health Journal, 12,* 172–79.

Essex, M. J., Klein, M. H., Cho, E., & Kalin, N. H. (2002). Maternal stress beginning in infancy may sensitize children to later stress exposure: Effects on cortisol and behavior. *Biological Psychiatry, 52,* 776–84.

Herman, J. (1992). *Trauma and Recovery: The aftermath of violence—From domestic abuse to political terror.* New York: Basic Books.

Ludermir, A. B., Lewis, G., Valongueiro, S.V., de Araújo, T. V. B., & Araya, R. (2010). Violence against women by their intimate partner during pregnancy and postnatal depression: A prospective cohort study. *Lancet, 376,* 903–10. Published online September 6, 2010 DOI:10.1016/S0140- 6736(10)60887-2.

Suglia, S. F., Enlow, M. B., Kullowatz, A., & Wright, R. J. (2009). Maternal intimate partner violence and increased asthma incidence in children: Buffering effects of supportive caregiving. *Arch Pediatr Adolesc Med, 163,* 244–50.

Walker, L. (1979). *The battered woman.* New York: Harper & Row.

Effects of War Trauma

Errebo, N. E. (1995). Object relations family therapy and PTSD: Family therapy with four generations of a Vietnam veteran's family. In D. K. Rhoades, M. R. Leaveck, & J. C. Hudson (Eds.), *The legacy of Vietnam veterans and their families: Survivors of war—Catalysts for changes*: Papers from the 1994 National Symposium (pp. 420–27). Washington, D.C.: Agent Orange Class Assistance Program.

Riggs, D. S., Byrne, C., Weathers, F., & Litz, B. (1998). The quality of intimate relationships of male Vietnam veterans: Problems associated with posttraumatic stress disorder. *Journal of Traumatic Stress, 11,* 87–101.

Chapter 9
Violence across the Life Span

Babinski, L. M., Hartsough, C. S., & Lambert, N. M. (1999). Childhood conduct problems, hyperactivity-impulsivity, and inattention as predictors of adult criminal activity. *Journal of Child Psychology and Psychiatry, 40*, 347–55.

Schaeffer, C. M., Petras, H., Ialongo, N., Poduska, J., & Kellam, S. (2003). Modeling growth in boys' aggressive behavior across elementary school: Links to later criminal involvement, conduct disorder, and antisocial personality disorder. *Developmental Psychology, 39*, 1020–35.

Substance Abuse

Brown, S. H., Gilman, S. G., Goodman, E. G., Adler-Tapia, R., & Freng, S. (in submission). Integrated trauma treatment: Combining EMDR and seeking safety.

Brown, S., Stowasser, J. E., & Shapiro, F. (2011). Eye movement desensitization and reprocessing (EMDR): Mental health-substance use. In D. B. Cooper (Ed.), *Intervention in mental health-substance use.* (pp. 165–93) Oxford: Radcliffe Publishing.

Kessler, R. C., Sonnega, A., Bromet, E., et al. (1995). Posttraumatic stress disorders in the National Comorbidity Survey. *Archives of General Psychiatry, 52*, 1048–60.

Najavits, L. M. (2002). *Seeking safety: A manual for PTSD and substance use treatment.* New York: Guilford.

Najavits, L. M., Weiss, R. D., & Shaw, S. R. (1999). A clinical profile of women with PTSD and substance dependence. *Psychology of Addictive Behaviors, 13*, 98–104.

Ouimette, P., & Brown, P. (Eds.) (2003). *Trauma and substance abuse: Causes, consequences and treatment of comorbid disorders.* Washington: American Psychological Association.

Ries, R. K., Miller, S. C., Fiellin, D. S., & Saitz, R. (2009). *Principles of addiction medicine (4th edition).* Philadelphia, PA: Lippincott.

Schneider Institute for Health Policy, Brandeis University for the Robert Wood Johnson Foundation (2001). *Substance abuse: The nation's number one health problem.* Princeton, NJ.

Shapiro, F., Vogelmann-Sine, S., & Sine, L. (1994). EMDR: Treating substance abuse and trauma. *Journal of Psychoactive Drugs, 26*, 379–91.

Zweben, J., & Yeary, J. (2006). EMDR in the treatment of addiction. *Journal of Chemical Dependency Treatment, 8*, 115–27.

Domestic Violence

Burke, J. G., Lee, L. C., & O'Campo, P. (2008). An exploration of maternal intimate partner violence experiences and infant general health and temperament. *Maternal Child Health Journal, 12*, 172–79.

Campbell, J. C., et al. (2003). Risk factors for femicide in abusive relationships: Results from a multisite case control study. *American Journal of Public Health, 93*, 1089–97.

Committee on the Judiciary United States Senate, 102nd Congress (1992). *Violence against women: A majority staff report.*

Dutton, D. G. (1998). *The abusive personality: Violence and control in intimate relationships.* New York: Guilford Press.

LaViolette, A. D., & Barnett, O. W. (2000). *It can happen to anyone: Why battered women stay.* Thousand Oaks, CA: Sage.

Ludermir, A. B., Lewis, G., Alves, S. V., de Araújo, T. V. B., & Araya, R. (2010). Violence against women by their intimate partner during pregnancy and postnatal depression: A prospective cohort study, *Lancet, 376,* 903–10, Published online September 6, 2010, DOI:10.1016/S0140-6736(10)60887-2.

Porges, S. W. (2007). The polyvagal perspective. *Biological Psychology, 74,* 116–43.

Rennison, C. M., & Welchans, S. (2000). *Bureau of Justice special report: Intimate partner violence.* Washington, DC: U.S. Department of Justice, Office of Justice Programs. Retrieved July 2, 2004, from http://www.ojp.usdoj.gov/ bjs/pub/pdf/ ipv.pdf.

Roberts, A. L., McLaughlin, K. A., Kerith, J., Conron, K. J., & Koenen, K. C. (2011). Adulthood stressors, history of childhood adversity, and risk of perpetration of intimate partner violence, *Am J Prev Med, 40,* 128–38.

Seligman, M. E. P. (1975). *Helplessness: On depression, development, and death.* San Francisco: W.H. Freeman.

Stowasser, J. (2007). EMDR and family therapy in the treatment of domestic violence. In F. Shapiro, F. Kaslow, & L. Maxfield (Eds.), *Handbook of EMDR and family therapy processes* (243–61). New York: Wiley.

Umhau, J. C., George, D. T., Reed, S., Petrulis, S. G., Rawlings, R., & Porges, S. W. (2002). Atypical autonomic regulation in perpetrators of violent domestic abuse. *Psychophysiology, 39,* 117–23.

Walker, L. (1979). *The battered woman.* New York: Harper & Row.

Child Sexual Abuse

Adler-Tapia, R., Settle, C., & Shapiro, F. (2012). Eye movement desensitization and reprocessing (EMDR) psychotherapy with children who have experienced sexual abuse and trauma. In P. Goodyear-Brown (Ed.), *The handbook of child sexual abuse: Identification, assessment and treatment.* (pp. 229–50) Hoboken, NJ: Wiley.

Finkelhor, D. (1994). Current information on the scope and nature of child sexual abuse. *Future Child, 4,* 31–53.

Hanson, R. K., Gordon, A., Harris, A. J. R., Marques, J. K., Murphy, W., Quinsey, V. L., & Seto, M. C. (2002). First report of the Collaborative Outcome Data Project on the effectiveness of psychological treatment for sexual offenders. *Sexual Abuse: A Journal of Research and Treatment, 14,* 169–94.

Jeperson, A. F., Lalumiere, M. L., & Seto, M. C. (2009). Sexual abuse history among adult sex offenders and non-sex offenders: A meta-analysis. *Child Abuse and Neglect, 33,* 179–92.

Marques, J. K., Wiederanders, M., Day, D. M., Nelson, C., & van Ommeren, A. (2005). Effects of a relapse prevention program on sexual recidivism: Final results from California's sex offender treatment and evaluation project (SOTEP). *Sexual Abuse: A Journal of Research and Treatment, 17,* 79–107.

McGrath, R. J., Cumming, G., Burchard, B., Zeoli, S., & Ellerby, L. (2009). *Current practices and trends in sexual abuse management. The safer society 2002 national survey.* Brandon, VT: Safer Society Foundation.

Pereda, N., Guilera, G., Forns, M., & Gómez-Benito, J. (2009). The prevalence of child sexual abuse in community and student samples: A meta-analysis. *Clin Psychol Rev. 29,* 328–38. Published online: March 5, 2009.

Ricci, R. J. (2006). Trauma resolution using eye movement desensitization and reprocessing with an incestuous sex offender, *Clinical Case Studies, 5,* 248–65.

Ricci, R. J., Clayton, C. A., & Shapiro, F. (2006). Some effects of EMDR on previously abused child molesters: Theoretical reviews and preliminary findings. *The Journal of Forensic Psychiatry & Psychology, 17*, 538–62.

van der Kolk, B. A. (1989). The compulsion to repeat the trauma: Re-enactment, revictimization, and masochism. *Psychiatric Clinics of North America, 12*, 389–411.

Walker, J. L., Carey, P. D., Mohr, N., Stein, D. J., & Seedat, S. (2004). Gender differences in the prevalence of childhood sexual abuse and in the development of pediatric PTSD. *Archives of Women's Mental Health, 7*, 111–21.

Trauma, Prison and Psychopathy

Caldwell, M., Skeem, J., Salekin, R., & Van Ryoboek, G. (2006). Treatment response of adolescent offenders with psychopathy features: A two-year follow-up. *Criminal Justice & Behavior, 33*, 571–96.

Chakhassi, F., de Ruiter, C., & Bernstein, D. (2010). Change during forensic treatment in psychopathic versus nonpsychopathic offenders. *Journal of Forensic Psychiatry and Psychology, 21*, 660–82.

Department of Policy and Legal Affairs. National Alliance on Mental Illness (n.d.). *A guide to mental illness and the criminal justice system: A systems guide for families and consumers.* Arlington, VA: National Alliance on Mental Illness.

Dyer, C. (2010). Re-offending rates are lower among offenders treated in secure hospitals than among mentally ill people held in prison. *British Medical Journal, 341*:c6447 doi: 10.1136/bmj.c6447.

Fazel, S., & Baillargeon, J. (2010). The health of prisoners. *Lancet, 377*, 956–65.

Heide, K. M., & Solomon, E. P. (2006). Biology, childhood trauma, and murder: Rethinking justice. *International Journal of Law and Psychiatry, 29*, 220–33.

James, D. J., & Glaze, L. E. (2006) *Mental health problems of prison and jail inmates.* Bureau of Justice Statistics Special Report, U.S. Department of Justice, Washington, D.C., NCJ 213600.

Kinsler, P. J., & Saxman, A. (2007). Traumatized offenders: Don't look now, but your jail's also your mental health center. *J Trauma Dissociation, 8*, 81–95.

Leon-Carrion, J., & Ramos, F. (2003). Blows to the head during development can predispose to violent criminal behaviour: Rehabilitation of consequences of head injury is a measure for crime prevention. *Brain Injury 15*, 207–16.

National GAINS Center for People with Co-Occurring Disorders in the Justice System (2001). *The prevalence of co-occurring mental health and substance use disorders in jails: Fact sheet series.* Delmar, NY: The National GAINS Center.

Skeem, J. L., Monahan, J., & Mulvey, E. P. (2002). Psychopathy, treatment involvement, and subsequent violence among civil psychiatric patients. *Law and Human Behavior, 26*, 577–603.

Solomon, E. P., & Heide, K. M. (2005). The biology of trauma: Implications for treatment. *Journal of Interpersonal Violence, 20*, 51–60.

van der Kolk, B. A. (1989). The compulsion to repeat the trauma: Re-enactment, revictimization, and masochism. *Psychiatric Clinics of North America, 12*, 389–411.

Chapters 10 and 11

Effects of Stress

Alfonso, J., Frasch, A. C., & Flugge, G. (2005). Chronic stress, depression and antidepressants: Effects on gene transcription in the hippocampus. *Rev Neurosci, 16*, 4356.

Champagne, F. A. (2010). Early adversity and developmental outcomes: Interaction between genetics, epigenetics, and social experiences across the life span. *Perspectives on Psychological Science, 5,* 564–74.

Epel, E. S., Blackburn, E. H., Lin, J., Dhabhar, F.S., et al. (2004). Accelerated telomere shortening in response to life stress. *PNAS, 101,* 17312–15.

McEwen, B. S. (2007). Physiology and neurobiology of stress and adaptation: Central role of the brain. *Physiol Rev, 87,* 873–904.

Ortega, F. B., Lee, D., Sui, X., Kubzansky, L. D., Ruiz, J. R., et al. (2010). Psychological well-being, cardiorespiratory fitness, and long-term survival. *Am J Prev Med, 39,* 440–48.

Sapolsky, R. M. (2004). Organismal stress and telomeric aging: An unexpected connection. *PNAS, 101,* 17323–24.

Simon, N. M., Smollera, J. W., McNamara, K. L., Master, R. S., et al. (2006). Telomere shortening and mood disorders: Preliminary support for a chronic stress model of accelerated aging. *Biological Psychiatry, 60,* 432–35.

Benefits of Stress Reduction, Meditation and Lifestyle Changes

Amen, D. (2010). *Change your brain, change your body.* New York: Harmony Books.

Bossini, L., Fagiolini, A., & Castrogiovanni, P. (2007). Neuroanatomical changes after eye movement desensitization and reprocessing (EMDR) treatment in post-traumatic stress disorder. *Journal of Neuropsychiatry and Clinical Neuroscience, 19,* 475–76.

Brown, K. W., Ryan, R. M., & Creswell, J. D. (2007). Mindfulness: Theoretical foundations and evidence for its salutary effects. *Psychological Inquiry, 18,* 211–37.

Davidson, R. J., Kabat-Zinn, J., Schumacher, J., Rosenkranz, M., Muller, D., Santorellie, S. F., et al. (2003). Alterations in brain and immune function produced by mindfulness meditation. *Psychosomatic Medicine, 65,* 564–70.

Doidge, N. (2007). *The brain that changes itself: Stories of personal triumph from the frontiers of brain science.* New York: Penguin.

Dunn, A. L., et al. (2005). Exercise treatment for depression: Efficacy and dose response. *American Journal of Preventive Medicine, 28,* 1–8.

Dusek, J. A., Out, H. H., Wohlhueter, A. L., Bhasin, M., Zerbini, L. F., et al. (2008). Genomic counter-stress changes induced by the relaxation response. *PLoS ONE 3*(7): e2576. doi:10.1371/journal.pone.0002576.

Jazayeri, S., et al. (2008). Comparison of therapeutic effects of omega-3 fatty acid eicosa-pentaenoic acid and fluoxetine, separately and in combination, in major depressive disorder. *Australian and New Zealand Journal of Psychiatry, 42,* 192–98.

Kabat-Zinn, J. (2005). *Coming to our senses.* New York: Hyperion.

Levine, S. (1991). *Guided meditations, explorations and healings.* New York: Anchor.

McEwen, B. S. (2007). Physiology and neurobiology of stress and adaptation: Central role of the brain. *Physiol Rev, 87,* 873–904.

Siegel, D. (2010). *Mindsight: The new science of personal transformation.* New York: Bantam.

Siegel, D. J. (2007). *The mindful brain: Reflection and attunement in the cultivation of well-being.* New York: W. W. Norton.

Servan-Schreiber, D. (2004). *The Instinct to Heal: Curing stress, anxiety and depression without drugs and without talk therapy.* New York: Rodale.

Anxiety, Imagery and Performance Enhancement

Burton, D. (1988). Do anxious swimmers swim slower? Reexamining the elusive anxiety-performance relationship. *Journal of Sports and Exercise Psychology, 10*, 45–61.

Barker, R. T., & Barker, S. B. (2007). The use of EMDR in reducing presentation anxiety. *Journal of EMDR Practice and Research, 1*, 100–108.

Foster, S., & Lendl, J. (1995). Eye movement desensitization and reprocessing: Initial applications for enhancing performance in athletes. *Journal of Applied Sport Psychology, 7* (Supplement), 63.

Foster, S., & Lendl, J. (2007). Eye movement desensitization and reprocessing: Four case studies of a new tool for executive coaching and restoring employee performance after setbacks. In R. R. Kilburg & R. C. Diedrich (Eds.), *The Wisdom of Coaching.* Washington, D.C: American Psychological Association Press.

Gould, D., & Tuffey, S. (1996). Zones of optimal functioning research: A review and critique. *Anxiety, Stress & Coping, 9*, 53–56.

Hall, C. (2001). Imagery in sport and exercise. In R. Singer, H. Hausenblas, & C. Janelle (Eds.), *Handbook of sport psychology* (pp. 529–49). New York: Wiley.

Murphy, S. M., Jowdy, D. P., & Durtschi, S. K. (1990). *Imagery Perspective Survey: U.S. Olympic Training Center.* Unpublished manuscript. U. S. Olympic Training Center.

Orlick, T., & Partington, J. (1988). Mental links to excellence. *The Sport Psychologist, 2*, 105–30.

Post, P. G., Wrisberg, C. A., & Mullins, S. (2010). A field test of the influence of pre-game imagery on basketball free throw shooting. *Journal of Imagery Research in Sport and Physical Activity, 5*, Available at: http://www.bepress.com/jirspa/vol5/iss1/art2 DOI: 10.2202/1932-0191.1042.

Szpunar, K. K., Watson, J. M., & McDermott, K. B. (2007). Neural substrates of envisioning the future. *PNAS, 104*, 642–47.

Wilson, G., Taylor, J., Gundersen, F., & Brahm, T. (2005). Intensity. In J. Taylor & G. Wilson (Eds.), *Applying sports psychology: Four perspectives* (pp. 33–49). Champaign, IL: Human Kinetics.

Stress Reduction and Performance Enhancement Procedures

Hays, K. F., & Brown, Jr., C. H. (2004). *You're on! Consulting for peak performance.* Washington, D.C.: American Psychological Association.

Lendl, J., & Foster, S. (2003). *EMDR: Performance enhancement for the workplace: A practitioner's guide.* Hamden, CT: EMDR-HAP.

Levine, S. (1991). *Guided meditations, explorations and healings.* New York: Anchor.

Lohr, B. A., & Scogin, F. (1998). Effects of self administered visuo-motor behavioral rehearsal on sports performance of collegiate athletes. *Journal of Sport Behavior. 21*, 206–18.

May, R. (2010). Sport performance interventions. In I. Weiner & W. E. Craighead (Eds.), *The Corsini encyclopedia of psychology* (4th edition). Vol. 4 (pp. 629–32). Hoboken, NJ: Wiley.

Orlick, T. (2007). *In pursuit of excellence.* Champaign, IL: Human Kinetics.

Shapiro, E. (2009). Four elements exercise for stress management. In M. Luber (Ed.), *EMDR scripted protocols.* New York: Springer.

Shapiro, F. (2001). *Eye movement desensitization and reprocessing: Basic principles, protocols and procedures* (2nd ed.). New York: Guilford Press.

Shapiro, F. (2006). *EMDR and new notes on adaptive information processing.* Camden, CT: EMDR Humanitarian Assistance Programs.

Global Outreach of EMDR

Abbasnejad, M., Mahani, K. N., & Zamyad, A. (2007). Efficacy of "eye movement desensitization and reprocessing" in reducing anxiety and unpleasant feelings due to earthquake experience. *Psychological Research, 9,* 104–17.

Aduriz, M. E., Bluthgen, C., & Knopfler, C. (2009). Helping child flood victims using group EMDR intervention in Argentina: Treatment outcome and gender differences. *International Journal of Stress Management, 16,* 138–53.

Brown, L. (2008). *Cultural competence in trauma therapy: Beyond the flashback.* Washington, DC: American Psychological Association.

EMDR Humanitarian Assistance Programs (2010). Accomplishments and efforts worldwide. http://www.emdrhap.org.

Fernandez, I., Gallinari, E., & Lorenzetti, A. (2004). A school-based EMDR intervention for children who witnessed the Pirelli building airplane crash in Milan, Italy. *Journal of Brief Therapy, 2,* 129–36.

Jarero, I., Artigas, L., Montero, M., & Lena, L. (2008). The EMDR integrative group treatment protocol: Application with child victims of a mass disaster. *Journal of EMDR Practice and Research, 2,* 97–105.

Konuk, E., Knipe, J., Eke, I., Yuksek, H., Yurtsever, A., & Ostep, S. (2006). The effects of EMDR therapy on post-traumatic stress disorder in survivors of the 1999 Marmara, Turkey, earthquake. *International Journal of Stress Management, 13,* 291–308.

Shapiro, F., & Solomon, R. (1995). Eye movement desensitization and reprocessing: Neurocognitive information processing. In G. Everley (Ed.), *Innovations in Disaster and Trauma Psychology, Vol. 1* (pp. 216–237). Elliot City, MD: Chevron Publishing.

Silver, S. M., Rogers, S., Knipe, J., & Colelli, G. (2005). EMDR therapy following the 9/11 terrorist attacks: A community-based intervention project in New York City. *International Journal of Stress Management, 12,* 29–42.

Solomon, R. M., & Rando, T. A. (2007). Utilization of EMDR in the treatment of grief and mourning. *Journal of EMDR Practice and Research, 1,* 109–17.

Sprang, G. (2001). The use of eye movement desensitization and reprocessing (EMDR) in the treatment of traumatic stress and complicated mourning: Psychological and behavioral outcomes. *Research on Social Work Practice, 11,* 300–320.

Wadaa, N. N., Zaharim, N. M., & Alqashan, H. F. (2010). The use of EMDR in treatment of traumatized Iraqi children. *Digest of Middle East Studies, 19,* 26–36.

Zaghrout-Hodali, M., Alissa, F., & Dodgson, P. W. (2008). Building resilience and dismantling fear: EMDR group protocol with children in an area of ongoing trauma. *Journal of EMDR Practice and Research, 2,* 106–13.

INDEX

Underscored references indicate tables.

A

Abandonment, fear of, 4–5, 12–14, 154, 249–52
Adaptive information processing, 20–23, 50
Adaptive resolution, 20–22
Addiction. *See* Drug use and addiction
ADHD, 174–76
Affect Scan technique, 78–79, 80, 86–88, 304
Air, in Four Elements technique, 261
Alcoholism. *See* Drug use and addiction
Antidepressants, 67
Antisocial behavior. *See also* Child abuse; Relationship problems; Sexual abuse
    domestic abuse, 190–95, 231–37
    drug use and addiction, 220–28, 277–80
    gangs, 229–31
    in kindergarten child, 216–20
    punishment for, 220
    resort to violence, 228–31
    sexual abusers, 237–44
    treatable nature of, 244–46
    understanding needed for, 215–16, 220, 226–27, 244, 246
Anxiety and fear. *See also* Lack of Control/Power; Lack of Safety/ Vulnerability; PTSD
    of abandonment, 4–5, 12–14, 154, 249–52
    about performance, 264–67, 268–71
    alternately tapping thighs for reducing, 56–57, 149–50
    of attention, 263–64
    Butterfly Hug for reducing, 57, 148–50, 304
    of crying, 46–47, 127–28
    of death, 170–72, 173–74
    of dogs and small animals, 128–29
    of driving, 126
    of flying, 47–52
    panic disorder, 73–75, 152–54, 156–57, 225–26, 248
    phobias, 120, 121–22, 124–29
    of public speaking, 7–9, 121
    of public transportation, 127
    of snakes, 128
    usefulness and naturalness of, 120
Asthma, 154–57
Attention Deficit Hyperactivity Disorder (ADHD), 174–76

B

Behavioral experiments, 125–26
Belly Breath technique, 118, 304
Bilateral stimulation with alternate tapping, 56–57, 149–50
Blame
    of addiction on lack of discipline, 224–25
    blaming the victim, 239–40, 241
    EMDR not about, 16
    self-blame, 135, 239, 241, 292–93
    tempering with understanding, 215–16, 244, 246
Body Changes technique, 266, 304
Body issues. *See also* Stress
    ADHD, 174–76
    appearance, 169
    asthma, 154–56
    brain/body connection, 157, 161–62, 166–67
    chronic pain, 172–73
    eating disorder, 12–14
    fear of death, 170–72, 173–74
    humiliation in childhood and, 167–69, 177–78
    migraines, 161–62
    mind/body connection, 172
    mistaken search for physical cures, 169–70
    panic disorder, 152–54, 156–57
    personal exploration of, 177, 178
    phantom limb pain, 158–61
    phantom pain, 162–63
    psychosomatic aspect of, 151–52
    range of sensations and effects, 156, 157
    sexual problems, 163–64
    shame about disfigurement, 176–77
    smell and sweating, 167–68
    somaticizing, 38

Bonding and attachment. *See also*
    Insecure attachment styles
    case histories, 95–97, 100–101, 102–3,
        104, 110–13
    causes of separation, 98–99
    father not bonding with baby, 99–100
    identifying Touchstone Memories,
        116–18
    insecure attachment styles, 101–5,
        111–13
    Lack of Safety/Vulnerability with,
        122–23
    mother not bonding with baby, 95–97,
        99, 100–101, 155–56
    panic disorder and, 154
    postpartum moods and, 100, 111
    relationship problems and, 182–85,
        186–88
    Responsibility issues with, 109–18
    secure attachment style, 102
    self-care, 118–19
    triangle with parents, 203–4
Brain. *See also* Unconscious mind
    adaptive resolution by, 20–22
    automatic responses by, 2–4
    body issues and, 157, 161–62, 166–67
    healing done by, 272
    hippocampus and PTSD, 29
    irrational responses by, 9
    multiple connections made by, 43
    panic disorder and, 153–54, 156–57
    psychosomatic issues, 151–52, 157
    unconscious based on workings of, 7
Breathing Shift technique, 55, 76, 80, 87,
    90, 304
Breathing techniques
    Belly Breath, 118, 304
    Breathing Shift, 55, 76, 80, 87, 90, 304
    Centering, 267–68, 304
    closing down disturbing memories, 149
Butterfly Hug technique, 57, 148–50, 304

C

C (Cognition) in TICES Log, 91
Cartoon Character technique, 58, 80, 90,
    149, 304
Centering technique, 267–68, 304
Child abuse. *See also* Insecure attachment
    styles
    case histories, 80–81, 82–83, 240–44
    disorganized attachment and, 104, 113

later relationship problems and,
    188–90, 197–202
Responsibility issues with, 113
sexual, 135–39, 197
sexual abusers, 237–44
Chronic pain, 172–73
Clinicians or therapists
    choosing, 306–7
    for depression, 107
    determining need for, 76, 94, 146–47
    needed for PTSD therapy, 32, 38
    partnership with, 303
    therapy and training resources, 307–8
Cognitive behavioral therapy (CBT),
    49–50
Control issues. *See* Lack of Control/Power
Crying, fear of, 46–47, 127–28
Culture and society
    compassion for others, 296–301
    death and grieving, 284–87
    disconnection from family, 276–80
    prejudice, 280–83
    religion and spirituality, 288–96

D

Death
    anger about, 286–87
    facing our own, 291–93
    fear of, 170–72, 173–74
    mourning, 284–86
Depression, 64–67, 106–7, 111, 146–47
Destructive behavior. *See* Antisocial
    behavior
Dismissive attachment style, 102–3, 111,
    183–84
Disorganized attachment style, 103–4,
    113
Domestic abuse, 190–95, 231–37
Drug Court Program, 221–22
Drug use and addiction, 220–28
    addictive behaviors, 227–28
    asking for help, 225
    discipline not enough for, 224–25
    disconnection from family and,
        277–80
    Drug Court Program, 221–22
    genetic predisposition to addiction,
        220
    panic attacks and, 225–26
    understanding needed for, 226–27
    untreated trauma and, 220–21, 228

E

E (Emotion) in TICES Log, 91
Earth, in Four Elements technique, 261
Eating disorder, 12–14
EMDR. *See also* Clinicians or therapists
  acronym explained, 24, 27–28
  CBT compared to, 49–51
  discovery of, 24–25
  effectiveness of, 6, 27
  eye movements used in, 30, 33,
    34–36
  inappropriate vs. appropriate reactions
    and, 47, 52
  initial investigation of, 25–26
  memory processing with, 31–38
  overview of process, 6, 310
  personality changes with, 39
  plateaus of processing, 136
  psychodynamic, compared to, 48
  PTSD study using, 26–27
  recognition by therapeutic community,
    26–27
  studies documenting, 27, 29, 30
  theories of why it works, 29–31
  therapy and training resources,
    307–8
  three steps in treatment, 269
  wide-ranging effects of, 28–29
EMDR-Humanitarian Assistance
  Program (HAP), 226, 298–301,
  309–10
Exercise, for stress relief, 257
Exposure therapy, 125–26

F

Faith. *See* Religion and spirituality
Family. *See* Relationship problems
Fear. *See* Anxiety and fear
Fire, in Four Elements technique, 262
Floatback technique
  Affect Scan with, 86–88
  exploring body issues, 177, 178
  identifying Touchstone Memories,
    117–18
  instructions for, 88
  returning to neutral after, 87
  tip for using, 143
  uses for, 304
Flying, fear of, 47–52
Four Elements technique, 260–62, 304
Future Template, 269–71, 304

G

Gangs, 229–31
Genetic issues
  attachment styles and, 105
  mental disorders and, 14–15, 71
  predisposition to addiction, 220
  reactivity to environmental stress and,
    97, 248
  relationship problems and, 181–82
  unprocessed memories triggering, 15,
    71
Grieving over death, 284–86
Guided visualization, 295, 305

H

Halo effect, 66, 283
HAP, 226, 298–301, 309–10
Hippocampus, 29
Horns effect, 283

I

I (Image) in TICES Log, 91
Insecure attachment styles
  case histories, 102–3, 104
  defined, 102
  dismissive attachment, 102–3, 111,
    183–84
  disorganized attachment, 103–4, 113
  identifying Touchstone Memories,
    116–18
  preoccupied attachment, 103, 112–13,
    186–87, 201–2
  relationship problems with, 182–85,
    186–88, 201–2
  Responsibility issues with, 109–18
  reversing the effects of, 104–5
  self-care for, 118–19
Internal locus of control, 143

L

Lack of Control/Power
  case histories, 16–17, 40, 139–40,
    143–44, 191–95
  domestic abuse and, 193–95, 231
  drivenness with, 144
  helplessness with, 143–44
  internal locus of control and, 143
  negative cognitions, 85, 143, 145
  positive cognitions countering, 85
  reducing anxiety and fear, 148–50
  stress and, 249–52

Lack of Control/Power *(cont.)*
    as third plateau of EMDR processing,
      136
    unable to choose, 16–17, 139–40
Lack of Safety/Vulnerability. *See also*
      Anxiety and fear; PTSD
    case histories, 12–14, 40, 64–67,
      121–23, 126–29, 142–43
    insecure attachment and, 122–23
    lack of caring due to, 140–41
    negative cognitions, 85, 124–25,
      141–42
    phobias, 120, 121–22, 124–29
    positive childhood example, 147–48
    positive cognitions countering, 85, 146
    secondary gain from, 129
    as second plateau of EMDR
      processing, 136
    self-care for, 146–50
    sexual abuse, 135–40
    wide variety of issues, 124
Lightstream technique, 179–80, 304

M

Marriage. *See* Relationship problems
Meditation, 288–90, 294–95, 304, 305
Memories, unprocessed. *See also*
    Touchstone Memories
    as cause of suffering, 11, 15
    childhood, as foundation of later
      symptoms, 41–43
    closing down disturbing memories, 149
    emotions, sensations, and beliefs
      stored with, 5, 22
    how EMDR works with, 31–38
    isolated from general memory
      networks, 22–23
    never too late to change, 62–63
    number responsible for current
      problems, 76, 89
    physical reactions due to, 89–90
    processed memories compared to,
      59–61
    processing, defined, 62
    PTSD due to, 10–11
    as triggers for disturbances, 70–72, 75
Memory retrieval, 76, 77–78, 106–7
Migraines, 161–62
Misattunement with child. *See* Insecure
    attachment styles
Mourning, 284–86

N

Negative cognitions, 80–89
    accessing memories for, 86–89
    categories of, 83–85, 108–9
    defined, 304
    descriptions versus, 82
    as how you feel about yourself, 82
    identifying, 81–86
    with Lack of Control/Power, 143, 145
    with Lack of Safety/Vulnerability,
      124–25, 141–42
    list of, 84–85
    with Responsibility issues, 113–15
    in TICES Log, 91
    unconscious processes revealed by, 86
    worst moments described by, 84
"No" and "Yes" experiment, 45, 47

O

Omega-3 fatty acids, 257

P

Pain. *See also* Body issues
    chronic, 172–73
    Lightstream technique for, 179–80
    migraines, 161–62
    phantom, 158–61, 162–63
    somaticizing, 38
Paint Can technique, 80, 90, 149, 304
Panic disorder, 73–75, 152–54, 156–57,
    225–26, 248
Personality, EMDR's affect on, 39
Personal Table, 302, 302–3
Phantom pain, 158–61, 162–63
Phobias, 120, 121–22, 124–29. *See also*
    Anxiety and fear
Positive cognitions, 84–85, 85–86, 146–47
Posttraumatic growth, 296
Prejudice, 280–83
Preoccupied attachment style, 103,
    112–13, 186–87, 201–2
Psychodynamic therapy, 48
Psychosomatic issues. *See* Body issues
PTSD, 129–35
    childhood events setting up, 133–35
    in combat veterans or first responders,
      10, 27, 62, 73–74, 92, 113,
      130–35, 207–9
    diagnosis of, 10
    after earthquake, 32–38
    EMDR study using, 26–27

hippocampus and, 29
Lack of Safety/Vulnerability with, 124–25
never too late to heal, 62–63
panic attacks with, 73–75
after plane crash, 245–46
range of symptoms with, 129–30, 131–32
symptoms with lesser experiences, 11, 14
therapist needed for exploring, 32, 38
unprocessed memories behind, 10–11
vicarious traumatization, 165–66
Public speaking, fear of, 7–9, 121

R

Rape, 139–40. *See also* Sexual abuse
Rapid eye movement (REM) sleep, 21, 28, 30
Rehearsing for success, 268–71
Relationship problems. *See also* Antisocial behavior
abuse in childhood and, 188–90, 197–202
attachment styles and, 182–85, 186–88
childhood trauma and, 12–14
closing off, 206–9
colliding networks, 39–40
disconnection from family, 276–80
domestic abuse, 190–95, 231–37
with family members, 210–12
fear of abandonment, 4–5
personal exploration of, 214
prevalence of, 181
Responsibility issues and, 205–6, 207–9
triangle with parents and, 203–4
Relationship suggestions
asking for help, 182, 202
communication skills, 185–86, 187, 214
knowing and communicating your triggers, 196
looking for the cause, 213
looking for trends, 196
making plans and agreements, 192–93, 195–96
practicing generosity, 213
staying open, 213–14
Time-Out plan, 196

Religion and spirituality, 288–96
facing death, 291–93
personal exploration of, 293–96
sinfulness, 290–91
spiritual disconnection, 288–90
REM sleep, 21, 28, 30
Responsibility issues (being defective)
attachment styles and, 109–18
case histories, 42–43, 63–64, 110–13, 272–73
as first plateau of EMDR processing, 136
identifying Touchstone Memories, 116–18
negative cognitions, 84, 113–15
positive cognitions countering, 84
preparations for dealing with, 116
relationship problems with, 205–6, 207–9
self-care for, 118–19
shame about disfigurement, 176–77
Revenge, 286–87
Roses are red..., 2–3, 66, 255

S

S (Sensation or SUD) in TICES Log, 91
Safe/Calm Place technique
basic technique, 53–55
bilateral stimulation with, 56–57
Breathing Shift technique with, 55, 57
closing down disturbing memories, 149
complex disorders not responding to, 76
connecting to positive feelings, 146
daily use of, 57
for expressing yourself, 206
for handling disturbances in life, 90
Lightstream technique with, 180
positive memory with, 54, 106–7
preparing for difficult situations, 119
returning to neutral with, 78, 80, 87
testing the effects of, 55–56
uses for, 305
Safety issues. *See* Lack of Safety/ Vulnerability
Secondary gain, 129
Self-blame
for sexual abuse, 135, 239, 241
for sickness, 292–93

Self-care
    for Lack of Safety/Vulnerability,
        146–50
    for Responsibility issues, 118–19
    for stress, 256–60, 265–71
Self-esteem issues. *See* Responsibility
        issues (being defective)
Sexual abuse
    blaming the victim, 239–40, 241
    case histories, 136–38, 139–40,
        197–200, 240–44
    child abuse, 135–39, 197
    child abusers, 237–44
    denial by abusers, 238
    getting help, 138–39
    plateaus of EMDR processing, 136
    rape, 139–40
    self-blame for, 135, 239, 241
Sexual performance problems,
        163–64
Shame. *See* Responsibility issues (being
        defective)
"Shoulds," 70, 87, 253–54
Sleep
    disturbed, 180
    REM, 21, 28, 30
Society. *See* Culture and society
Somaticizing, 38
Spiral technique, 107–8, 119, 149, 305
Spirituality. *See* Religion and spirituality
Stress
    anniversary of events and, 255–56
    control issues and, 253–54
    in family and relationships, 249–52
    Four Elements for reducing, 260–62
    genetic issues and, 97, 248
    panic disorder with, 248
    self-awareness reducing, 257–59
    self-care for, 256–60, 265–71
    Timeline for understanding, 259–60
    well-being vs. alleviating, 273–74
    in workplace, 252–54, 263–67,
        272–73
Subjective Units of Distress (SUD) scale,
        75–76, 78, 91, 305
Substance abuse. *See* Drug use and
        addiction

T

T (Trigger) in TICES Log, 91
Tapping thighs alternately, 56–57, 149–50
Techniques and tools, 304–5. *See also*
        specific kinds
Therapists. *See* Clinicians or therapists
TICES Log, 91–94, 257, 302–3, 305
Timeline, 259–60, 302–3, 305
Time-Out plan, 195–96
Touchstone List
    creating for recent upsets, 78
    defined, 305
    Floatback technique with, 87, 88–89
    job performance and, 266
    negative cognitions in, 83
    TICES Log for constructing, 302–3
Touchstone Memories. *See also*
        Memories, unprocessed
    current situations triggering, 78
    defined, 75, 305
    determining when professional help is
        needed, 76
    identifying for Responsibility issues,
        116–18
    many experiences tied to, 65
    network of memories connected to, 90
Triangle with parents, 203–4

U

Unconscious mind, 3, 7, 9, 86
Unprocessed memories. *See* Memories,
        unprocessed

V

Vulnerability. *See* Lack of Safety/
        Vulnerability

W

Water, in Four Elements technique,
        261–62
Water Hose technique, 59, 90, 305
Wet Eraser technique, 59, 90, 305

Y

"Yes" and "No" experiment, 45, 47